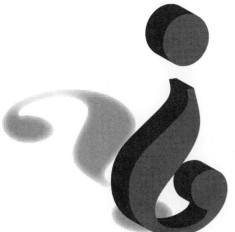

W0006411

Problem-Based Medical Spanish

William Joaquin Adamás-Rappaport, MD
Associate Professor of Surgery and Anatomy
Department of Surgery and Anatomy
University of Arizona Medical School;
Physician
Compass Health Care
Tucson, Arizona

Oscar Beita Quesada, MD, MPH
Clinical Assistant Professor
Department of Family and Community Medicine;
Assistant Director, Office of Outreach and
    Multicultural Affairs
The University of Arizona College of Medicine
Tucson, Arizona

Mara Gricel SantaMaria
First-Year Medical Student
College of Medicine
University of Arizona
Tucson, Arizona

Bardo Daniel Padilla Verlarde, MA
Instructional Faculty, Languages
Pima County Community College
Tucson, Arizona

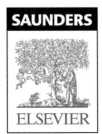

SAUNDERS

ELSEVIER

SAUNDERS
ELSEVIER

1600 John F. Kennedy Blvd.
Ste 1800
Philadelphia, PA 19103-2899

ISBN: 978-1-4160-3658-6

Notice

Knowledge and best practice in this field are constantly changing. As new research and experience broaden our knowledge, changes in practice, treatment, and drug therapy may become necessary or appropriate. Readers are advised to check the most current information provided (i) on procedures featured or (ii) by the manufacturer of each product to be administered to verify the recommended dose or formula, the method and duration of administration, and contraindications. It is the responsibility of the practitioner, relying on his or her own experience and knowledge of the patient, to make diagnoses, to determine dosages and the best treatment for each individual patient, and to take all appropriate safety precautions. To the fullest extent of the law, neither the Publisher nor the Author assumes any liability for any injury and/or damage to persons or property arising out or related to any use of the material contained in this book.

The Publisher

Library of Congress Cataloging-in-Publication Data
Adamás-Rappaport, William.
  Problem-based medical Spanish / William Joaquin Adamás-Rappaport, with the collaboration of Oscar Beita Quesada ... [et al.].—1st ed.
    p. ; cm.
  Includes bibliographical references and index.
  ISBN 978-1-4160-3658-6
  1. Spanish language—Conversation and phrase books (for medical personnel) 2. Medicine—Phrases—English. 3. Medicine—Phrases—Spanish. 4. Physical Examination—Phrases—English. 5. Physical Examination—Phrases—Spanish. 6. Problem-Based Learning—Phrases—English. 7. Problem-Based Learning—Phrases—Spanish. I. Title.

PQ4120.M3A63 2008
468.3′42102461—dc22

2007022796

Acquisitions Editor: Jim Merritt
Developmental Editor: Andrea Vosburgh
Design Direction: Karen O'Keefe Owens

Printed in the United States of America

Last digit is print number 9 8 7 6 5 4 3 2 1

Preface

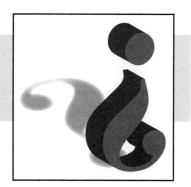

Problem-Based Medical Spanish is specifically designed for future health care professionals who require a more profound understanding of medical Spanish than is offered by most medical Spanish books on the market today. Specifically, the presentations are case-based as well as organ system–based. Because of the in-depth nature of the cases presented, we chose in this book to focus on urgent and emergent situations that bring patients to the emergency room, urgent care, or clinic.

The format follows the same pattern for each section. First, a patient is presented with a specific chief complaint—for example, chest pain. The initial step is to review anatomy. History and physical exam follow. Next, the discussion moves to differential diagnosis, then to workup and follow-up. The section concludes with a review of the pathophysiology of the disease process. Following the case presentations, each chapter includes sections on vocabulary and grammar as well as a brief discussion about cultural issues. Each chapter intends to build on the those prior to it in terms of grammar.

We chose five broad topics for this book: abdominal pain, chest pain, gynecologic and obstetric emergencies, pediatric emergencies, and urologic emergencies. The majority of urgent and emergent presentations in the emergency room, urgent-care setting, and clinic will likely fall under these headings. If a patient falls outside these main headings—for example, a patient with a fractured leg—the format of questions can be adjusted to conduct a logical history and physical exam and thereby arrive at a logical differential diagnosis. In addition, work-up and follow-up can also be reconstructed based on the presentations presented.

It is suggested that the reader have at least two years of Spanish, preferably at the college level, before tackling this book, although a highly motivated person might do well with just one year. Learning any language is a process, and practice is of the utmost importance. There are innumerable opportunities to practice your Spanish, not just in the medical setting. Don't be embarrassed if your pronunciation is not perfect or if you use the wrong words. The biggest obstacle I see to students and people in general speaking Spanish is an embarrassment at not being perfect. Remember that it is about communication with your patient. Your Spanish-speaking patients deeply appreciate the effort you are making to communicate with them. When you first start out you can have an interpreter in the room when you are talking with your patients; later, when you become proficient, you can conduct the interview by yourself.

Each copy of the book includes two CDs that contain audio files of the dialogues and other exercises to practice listening and speaking.

William Joaquin Adamás-Rappaport, MD

Contents

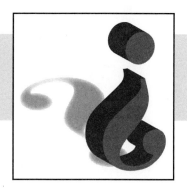

1 Abdominal Pain

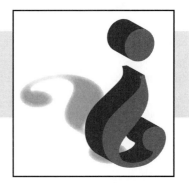

INTRODUCTION

Abdominal pain is one of the most common chief complaints of patients presenting to their physician. With a careful, focused history and physical exam a differential diagnosis is formed allowing a logical workup to proceed.

The keys are to:

(1) Differentiate between surgical (conditions requiring surgery, such as appendicitis) versus non-surgical causes (medical causes of abdominal pain, such as constipation or side effects of certain medications).

(2) Determine if the patient needs hospitalization (suspected appendicitis) or if the patient can be sent home with medication and have the workup performed as an outpatient (duodenal ulcer).

(3) Determine if the patient requires emergency surgery (perforated ulcer) or if a workup can be performed electively as an outpatient (suspected gallstones with mild abdominal discomfort, termed biliary colic).

ANATOMY

Intra-abdominal organs and common pains related to them are discussed in Table 1-1 and Figure 1-1. Figure 1-2 illustrates the correlation between anatomy and pathologic condition.

PHYSIOLOGIC CONSIDERATIONS OF ABDOMINAL PAIN

Abdominal pain arising from a pathologic intra-abdominal condition is divided into visceral and parietal pain. Visceral pain is dull and poorly localized. It is often described as dull, aching, cramping, and/or burning. This type of pain involves the visceral peritoneum, which covers all the visceral organs such as the liver, spleen, stomach, duodenum, small and large intestine, gallbladder, appendix, etc. Inflammation, if confined to the visceral peritoneum, will

Table 1-1. Anatomic Correlation of Abdominal Pain with Location ■ Correlación Anatómica del Dolor Abdominal con su Ubicación

Right Upper Quadrant (RUQ)	Epigastric Region	Left Upper Quadrant (LUQ)	Cuadrante Superior Derecho (CSD)	Región Epigástrica	Cuadrante Superior Izquierdo (CSI)
• Diaphragm • Duodenum • Liver • Head of pancreas • Gallbladder • Kidney • Right lower lobe of the lung	• Duodenum • Body pancreas • Common bile duct • Stomach • Esophagus • Aorta	• Spleen • Stomach • Diaphragm • Left lower lobe of the lung • Tail of pancreas • Kidney	• Diafragma • Duodeno • Hígado • Cabeza del páncreas • Vesícula biliar • Riñón • Lóbulo inferior derecho del pulmón	• Duodeno • Cuerpo del páncreas • Conducto biliar común • Estómago • Esófago • Aorta	• Bazo • Estómago • Diafragma • Lóbulo inferior izquierdo del pulmón • Cola del páncreas • Riñón
Right Lower Quadrant (RLQ)	**Suprapubic Region**	**Left Lower Quadrant (LLQ)**	**Cuadrante Inferior Derecho (CID)**	**Región Suprapúbica**	**Cuadrante Inferior Izquierdo (CII)**
• Cecum • Appendix • Ureter • Iliac artery • Ovary and fallopian tube	• Bladder • Uterus • Aorta	• Sigmoid colon • Ureter • Ovary and fallopian tube • Iliac artery	• Ciego • Apéndice cecal • Uréter • Arteria iliaca • Ovario y trompa de Falopio	• Vejiga • Útero • Aorta	• Colon sigmoides • Uréter • Ovario y trompa de Falopio • Arteria iliaca

Figure 1-1. Intra-abdominal organs in English and Spanish.

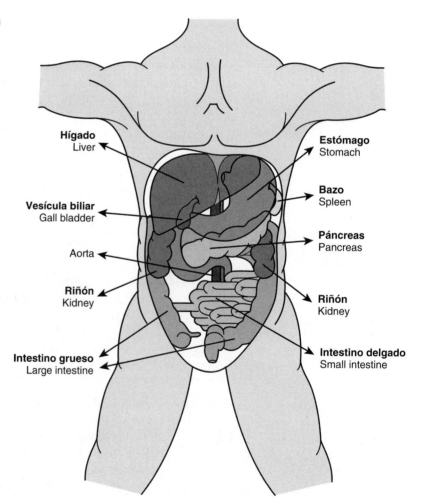

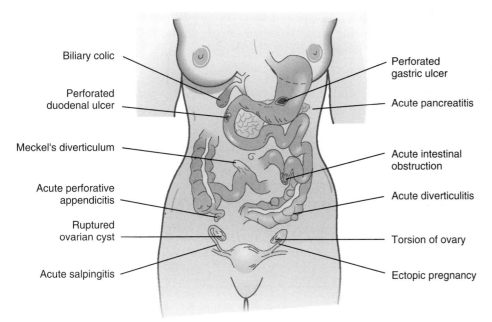

Figure 1-2. Common causes of abdominal pain. (From Townsend C: *Sabiston Textbook of Surgery*, ed 17, Philadelphia, Saunders, 2004.)

Biliary colic

Perforated duodenal ulcer

Meckel's diverticulum

Acute perforative appendicitis

Ruptured ovarian cyst

Acute salpingitis

Perforated gastric ulcer

Acute pancreatitis

Acute intestinal obstruction

Acute diverticulitis

Torsion of ovary

Ectopic pregnancy

present with this type of pain. This type of pain is also seen with distention of visceral organs such as the gallbladder or intestine (Fig. 1-3). The visceral nerve fibers travel with the sympathetic nerves and enter the spinal cord often at more than one level, thus producing a pain that is poorly localized. Parietal pain is localized and much more intense in terms of quality. These nerves follow the somatic nerve fibers and enter the cord at one level, producing a localized, intense pain. This involves inflammation of the parietal peritoneum, which lines the innermost layer of the anterior, lateral, and inferior abdominal wall. It is also the layer that overlies the retroperitoneal structures such as the kidney, pancreas, and aorta.

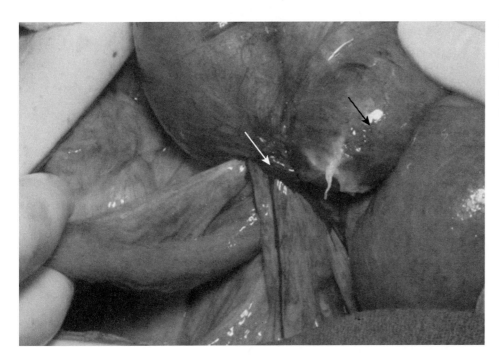

Figure 1-3. Small bowel obstruction from adhesion from prior surgery (*white arrow*). Note dilated proximal small bowel (*black arrow*) and collapsed distal small bowel.

Thus the pain of early appendicitis is due to distention of the appendix (visceral pain) producing a poorly localized pain in the periumbilical region, but as the disease progresses and involves the parietal peritoneum, it becomes localized to the right lower quadrant (RLQ).

CASE 1: CHOLECYSTITIS

CHIEF COMPLAINT

A young female patient presents with right upper quadrant pain of 12 hours' duration.

FOCUSED HISTORY

A focused history is concentrated on the chief complaint. In contrast, a complete history is much more extensive. The former is most often used in the emergency room or in clinic when dealing with a potentially serious condition that may require hospitalization and possibly surgery. The latter is often performed in an elective non-urgent situation such as a yearly exam.

When dealing with pain in any patient, whether it is abdominal, chest, bone, etc., the following questions should be asked in regard to the pain. Based on these questions, we often have a really good idea of what our patient has prior to beginning the physical exam.

1. **Quality**: How severe is it? Is it sharp, dull, burning, etc.? Has it changed? Is it getting worse?
2. **Location**: In the case of abdominal pain, this is crucial (always remember your anatomy); does the pain move or radiate? Has it changed location?
3. **Duration**: When did it begin?
4. Is it **Constant** or does it **Come** and **Go**?
5. **Precipitating Factors**: What makes it worse?
6. **Relieving Factors**: What makes it better?
7. **Associated Symptoms**: Nausea, vomiting, sweating, etc.

	English	Spanish Formal	Spanish Informal
	Ms. Martínez, my name is Tom Parsons, I am a third year medical student working with Doctor Johnson. I will be asking you some questions regarding your problem.	Señorita Martínez, mi nombre es Tom Parsons. Soy estudiante de medicina de tercer año y estoy trabajando con el Doctor Johnson. Le voy a hacer unas preguntas sobre su problema de salud.	Señorita Martínez, me llamo Tom Parsons. Soy estudiante de medicina de tercer año. Trabajo con el Doctor Johnson. Voy a hacerle unas preguntas.
Q.	How old are you?	¿Qué edad tiene?	¿Cuántos años tiene?
A.	I am thirty-five years old.	Tengo treinta y cinco años.	Treinta y cinco.
Q.	When did the pain start?	¿Cuándo comenzó el dolor?	¿Cuándo empezó el dolor?
A.	It began early in the morning some time.	Me comenzó temprano por la mañana.	Temprano en la mañana.

	English	Spanish Formal	Spanish Informal
Q.	Where is the pain located? Can you point to where it hurts?	¿Dónde le duele? ¿Me puede mostrar dónde le duele?	Enséñeme dónde le duele.
A.	It is located on the right side under the ribs, high up.	Me duele del lado derecho, debajo de las costillas, para arriba.	Aquí, en el lado derecho, debajo de las costillas.
Q.	How would you describe it (sharp, dull, burning, cramping)?	¿Cómo describiría el dolor? (agudo, sordo, quemante, retortijón).	¿Cómo es el dolor?
A.	It began as a dull pain but now it is sharp.	Comenzó como un dolor sordo pero ahora es agudo.	Me comenzó a doler por toda la panza, pero ahora solo me duele aquí (*debajo de las costillas*).
Q.	Is it constant or does it come and go?	¿Es constante o intermitente (*le va y le viene*)?	¿Es todo el tiempo o le pega y se le quita?
A.	Now it is constant. In the beginning it came and went.	Ahora es constante (*lo tengo todo el tiempo*). Al principio me pegaba y después se me quitaba.	Ahora me duele todo el tiempo. Antes me pegaba y después se me quitaba.
Q.	Does it move anywhere?	¿Se le mueve para alguna otra parte?	¿Se le mueve para algún lado?
A.	It moves around to the back on the right side. (Patient points to her scapula.)	Se me mueve para el lado derecho de la espalda (paciente señala la escápula).	Se me va para la paleta del lado derecho.
Q.	What makes it better?	¿Con qué se le alivia (*se le quita*)?	¿Hay algo que se lo quita?
A.	If I move around it hurts. If I lie still it doesn't hurt so badly.	Si me muevo, me duele. Si me acuesto y me quedo quieta, no me duele tanto.	Me duele cuando me muevo. Si me quedo quieta, no me duele.
Q.	Have you ever had this pain before?	¿Ha tenido este dolor anteriormente?	¿Ha tenido este dolor antes?
A.	I have had this pain often in the past year, mostly after eating, but it always went away.	Sí, he tenido este dolor varias veces en el último año, casi siempre después de comer, pero siempre se me había aliviado.	Varias veces después de comer, pero siempre se me había quitado.
Q.	Have you had nausea, vomiting, fever, or chills?	¿Ha tenido nausea, vómitos, fiebre o escalofríos?	¿Ha tenido ganas de vomitar, calentura o escalofríos?
A.	I vomited twice and am nauseated. I do feel warm. I haven't had chills.	Vomité dos veces y ahora tengo ganas (*nauseas*). Me siento afiebrada (*con fiebre*). No he tenido escalofríos (*calofríos*).	Arrojé dos veces y ahora tengo ganas. Siento como si tuviera calentura.
Q.	Do you drink alcohol or do you use any drugs?	¿Toma usted alcohol o usa drogas?	¿Toma licor o usa drogas?
A.	On weekends I have a couple of beers, but haven't drunk recently.	Los fines de semana me tomo un par de cervezas, pero no he tomado últimamente.	Los fines de semana me tomo un par de cervezas.
Q.	Do you take any medications?	¿Está tomando alguna medicina?	¿Toma alguna medicina?
A.	I took Motrin for the pain one hour ago.	Me tomé una Motrin para el dolor hace una hora.	Me tomé una pastilla para el dolor hace un rato.
Q.	Have you noted your urine turn darker, like Coca Cola?	¿Ha notado que la orina se le pone más oscura, como Coca Cola?	¿Ha orinado oscuro, como Coca Cola?
A.	No, it is clear.	No, es clara (*normal*).	No.
Q.	Have you noted your skin turning yellow?	¿Ha notado que la piel se le ha puesto amarilla?	¿Se le ha puesto amarilla la piel?
A.	No, it has not changed.	No, no ha cambiado.	No.

	English	Spanish Formal	Spanish Informal	Continued
Q.	When was your last period? (It is important to ask any young woman who presents with abdominal pain questions regarding the possibility of pregnancy. Ectopic pregnancy [pregnancy outside of the uterus] is a life-threatening emergency and may present initially with abdominal pain [usually lower abdomen].)	¿Cuándo fue su última menstruación?	¿Cuándo tuvo la última regla?	
A.	My last period was two weeks ago.	Mi última menstruación fue hace dos semanas.	Hace dos semanas.	
Q.	Are you active sexually, and if so, do you use some form of contraception?	¿Tiene relaciones sexuales? y de ser así, ¿qué método anticonceptivo usa para protegerse?	¿Está teniendo relaciones sexuales? ¿Qué hace para protegerse?	
A.	Yes, I take birth control pills.	Sí, tomo pastillas anticonceptivas.	Sí, tomo pastillas.	
Q.	Is there any burning on urination?	¿Le arde cuando orina?	¿Siente quemazón al orinar?	
A.	No, I haven't noticed any problem urinating.	No, no he notado ningún problema al orinar.	No.	
Q.	Have you had any recent travel outside the United States?	¿Ha viajado recientemente a algún lugar fuera de los Estados Unidos?	¿Ha viajado al extranjero recientemente?	
A.	No, I have not traveled outside the United States in the past year.	No, no he viajado fuera de los Estados Unidos en el último año.	No en el último año.	

FOCUSED PHYSICAL EXAM

The physical exam of the abdomen is crucial in the diagnosis of abdominal pain. Inspection of the abdomen, auscultation of bowel sounds, percussion, and palpation to determine the location and degree of tenderness constitute a complete abdominal exam. In the focused exam, one also examines the lungs and the heart. If indicated (i.e., lower abdominal pain in a female patient), a pelvic exam would be performed. Cardiac disease such as an inferior myocardial infarction may present as upper abdominal pain, and lower lobe pneumonia may also present with abdominal pain, thus stressing the importance of the cardiac and pulmonary exam. A check for hernias and a genitourinary exam are important especially in children, where a torsion (twisting of the testicle) may present with abdominal pain. If the bowel is trapped inside a hernia (incarceration), then abdominal pain and vomiting might be the predominant symptoms. Finally, a rectal exam is performed if clinically indicated (i.e., a patient who presents with lower abdominal pain or rectal bleeding and abdominal pain). A rectal exam will possibly allow the palpation of a rectal tumor if present and will allow the testing of stool on the gloved finger for blood (stool guiac test).

English	Spanish Formal	Spanish Informal
Ms. Martínez, I need to perform a physical exam. I will be listening to your heart and lungs and will examine your	Srta. Martínez, ahora necesito hacerle un examen físico. Le voy a escuchar el corazón y los pulmones y a examinarle el	Srta. Martínez, ahora la voy a examinar. Le voy a escuchar el corazón y los pulmones, y a tocarle la panza. Voy a salir un

English	Spanish Formal	Spanish Informal
abdomen. I will step out while you change into a gown. You may leave your underwear on. I will return shortly.	abdomen. Voy a salir del cuarto por un momento para que usted se ponga esta bata. Se puede dejar la ropa interior. Voy a regresar en un momento.	momento. Mientras vuelvo, quítese la ropa y póngase esta bata. Se puede quedar con la ropa interior.
Upon returning: I am going to take your blood pressure, temperature, pulse, and respirations first.	*Al regresar*: Primero le voy a tomar la presión arterial, la temperatura, el pulso y la frecuencia respiratoria.	*Al regresar*: Le voy a tomar la presión, la temperatura, el pulso y la frecuencia respiratoria.
Next I need to listen to your heart. I am going to listen to your lungs. (It is very important to describe to the patient each exam you are performing.)	Después le voy a escuchar el corazón. Le voy a escuchar los pulmones. (Es muy importante describirle al paciente cada examen que le va a realizar.)	Después le voy a escuchar el corazón y los pulmones.
Next I will examine your abdomen. I will press very softly. Please tell me if it hurts even slightly. (Always start away from the area of maximal tenderness and save this area until last in the abdominal exam. If this part of the abdomen is examined first, then the patient will tighten up his or her abdominal wall muscles [called guarding] and an accurate exam will be difficult.)	Ahora le voy a examinar el abdomen. Lo voy a apretar suavemente. Por favor dígame si le duele aunque sea poco. (Siempre hay que comenzar lejos del área más sensible, y dejar esta área para el final del examen abdominal. Si esta parte del abdomen se examina primero, el paciente va a contraer los músculos de la pared abdominal [llamado defensa] y se hace difícil realizar un examen preciso.)	Ahora le voy a examinar la panza. ¿Le duele cuando la toco?
Following the exam: Please get dressed and I will return shortly and we will discuss the possible causes of your abdominal pain.	*Después del examen*: Vístase, por favor, yo regresaré en un momento para hablar con usted sobre las posibles causas de su dolor abdominal.	*Después del examen*: Póngase la ropa, por favor. Cuando vuelva, vamos a conversar sobre lo que puede ser la causa de su dolor de panza.

PHYSICAL EXAM RESULTS

The following are the physical exam findings:

1. **Vital Signs (VS)**: Blood pressure (BP): 110/70; Pulse: 110 per minute; Respiratory rate (RR): 18 per minute; Temperature: 38.0° C.

2. **Lungs**: Clear

3. **Heart**: Rapid regular rate, normal S1 and S2, no S3 or S4, no murmur

4. **Abdomen**: The abdomen is mildly distended. Bowel sounds are present. Moderate tenderness is present in the right upper quadrant (RUQ). There is voluntary guarding present in the RUQ. The liver is not enlarged.

We will focus on the abdominal exam (the cardiac and pulmonary exam will be covered elsewhere in the book).

Abdominal distention is a non-specific finding. Any time there is intra-abdominal inflammation, i.e., appendicitis, cholecystitis, etc., the bowel stops normal peristalsis (termed ileus). Distention can also be seen in bowel obstruction where there is a blockage in the intestine from cancer or scar tissue from prior surgery. Finally, distention can result from fluid in the abdominal cavity as is seen in patients with ascites from cirrhosis of the liver.

Bowel sounds are the sounds made primarily from the peristalsis of the small intestine. Thus they are heard best over the lower mid-abdomen. The movement of fluid against the walls of the intestine during peristalsis produces these sounds. They may be diminished or absent when peritonitis or diffuse inflammation is present within the abdomen; such is the case of a perforated ulcer and peritonitis.

The location of the point of maximal tenderness is crucial. In the above case one must think about the anatomy, i.e., those structures present in the RUQ.

Guarding is a crucial finding in the exam of the abdomen. There are two types of guarding: voluntary and involuntary. Guarding refers to the consistency of the abdominal wall musculature. In a normal exam, the muscle is soft to palpation. When inflammation or distention of the abdominal viscera is present, the patient will tense the muscles voluntarily (voluntary guarding) when the examiner palpates over the affected area. However, with continued gentle pressure the muscles will relax. Involuntary guarding is highly significant and implies parietal peritoneal inflammation. There is rigidity throughout inspiration and expiration and the patient cannot relax the muscles. This may be seen with a perforated ulcer where the acid spills into the peritoneal cavity and diffuse rigidity is noted, or in advanced appendicitis, where the inflammation has reached the parietal peritoneum of the abdominal wall. Involuntary guarding is often an indication that surgical intervention will be required.

Following our history and physical exam, we form a differential diagnosis. Based on the possible etiologies of the patient's pain, we make a list with the most to least probable causes. This will allow a logical workup. Think anatomically. Incorporate your physical findings along with your history. This list will guide the subsequent workup.

DIFFERENTIAL DIAGNOSIS

English	Spanish Formal	Spanish Informal
• Cholecystitis	• Colecistitis	• Inflamación de la vesícula
• Hepatitis	• Hepatitis	• Hepatitis
• Pancreatitis	• Pancreatitis	• Inflamación del páncreas
• Peptic ulcer disease	• Enfermedad de la úlcera péptica	• Úlcera del estómago
• Pyelonephritis (infection in the kidney)	• Pielonefritis (infección del riñón)	• Inflamación de los riñones
Ms. Martínez, based on your history and the physical exam, I believe your problem is due to an inflammation in your gallbladder. This is most often caused by gallstones. We have to perform some tests of your blood and urine and obtain an x-ray of the gallbladder, called an ultrasound, to confirm the diagnosis and rule out other causes of your pain.	Srta. Martínez, en base a la historia y al examen físico, yo creo que lo que usted tiene es una inflamación de la vesícula biliar. Esto casi siempre se debe a piedras (*cálculos*) en la vesícula. Ahora tenemos que hacerle exámenes de sangre y orina y una radiografía de la vesícula, que se llama ultrasonido, para confirmar el diagnóstico y descartar otras causas de dolor.	Srta. Martínez, creo que usted tiene piedras en la vesícula. Tenemos que hacerle unos exámenes de sangre y orina, y un ultrasonido para confirmar el diagnóstico y descartar que no sea otra cosa.

Now comes a crucial decision. Does this patient need to be hospitalized or can you work this patient up as an outpatient?

This patient needs to be admitted to the hospital due to the following: she is vomiting and is nauseated and this will cause dehydration. In addition, the pain is getting worse and it is unremitting; she is tachycardic (rapid pulse); she has fever, which can be a sign of systemic infection or inflammation; and finally she has tenderness and voluntary guarding, again a sign of inflammation. The first step is starting intravenous fluids to restore the intravascular volume, which is depleted due to vomiting and nausea. Also, with any inflammation, capillaries become more permeable and fluid is lost to the surrounding space. Thus the patient with intra-abdominal inflammation suffers from intravascular volume depletion. Antibiotics are ordered for the suspected infection in the gallbladder, i.e., cholecystitis. *E. coli* is the most common infecting organism in cholecystitis, thus your choice of an antibiotic must cover these bacteria. The patient is then taken to radiology for an ultrasound, which is the most sensitive test (95% sensitive) for diagnosing gallstones and accompanying inflammation (cholecystitis).

English	Spanish Formal	Spanish Informal
Ms. Martínez, we will need to admit you into the hospital to give you fluids through your vein and antibiotics since we suspect an infection in your gallbladder. This can be serious if not treated. We will know much more after the tests come back.	Srta. Martínez, necesitamos internarla (*ingresarla*) en el hospital para ponerle suero intravenoso y antibióticos. Sospechamos que usted tiene una infección de la vesícula biliar. Puede ser grave si no recibe tratamiento. Vamos a tener más información cuando tengamos los resultados de las pruebas de laboratorio.	Srta. Martínez, la vamos a internar para ponerle suero y antibióticos. Creemos que tiene una infección de la vesícula. Puede ser grave si no le damos tratamiento. Estamos esperando los resultados de las pruebas que le hicimos para saber más.

TEST RESULTS

- The ultrasound shows gallstones, thickening of the gallbladder wall, and a normal common bile duct (Fig. 1-4).
- White blood cell (WBC) count: 15,000 (elevated)
- Serum sodium, potassium, chloride, glucose, blood urea nitrogen: within normal limits (WNL).
- Hemoglobin: 13.4; Hematocrit: 41% (WNL)
- Amylase: 125 (WNL)
- Liver function tests (LFTs):
  - AST: WNL
  - ALT: WNL
- Bilirubin: WNL
- Alkaline phosphatase: WNL
- Urine analyses: no WBCs, occasional bacteria seen
- Urine pregnancy: Negative

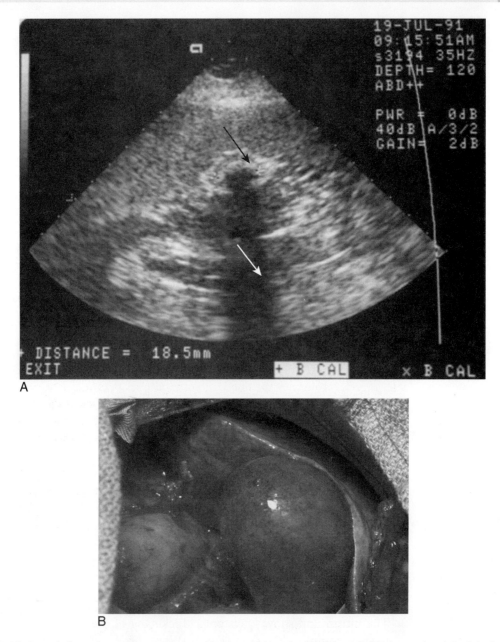

Figure 1-4. A, Ultrasound of a patient with acute cholecystitis. Note thickened gallbladder wall (*black arrow*) and the "shadowing" (*white arrow*) due to gallbladder stones. **B,** Intra-operative findings of acute cholecystitis due to obstruction of the cystic duct by a gallstone. Note acutely distended and inflamed gallbladder.

What Do These Tests Tell You?

A normal serum amylase, an enzyme that is produced in the pancreas, in most cases rules out pancreatitis. In pancreatitis, due to inflammation of the pancreas, amylase is released in the circulation and an elevated serum amylase is seen. In most cases, a serum lipase should also be checked, since it is more specific for pancreatic inflammation than amylase. The two most common causes of pancreatitis are alcohol, which directly damages the pancreatic acinar cells, and gallstones (cholelithiasis). If the gallstones are small, they may move through the cystic duct and pass through into the ampulla of Vater, causing bile to reflux up the pancreatic duct, injuring the pancreas and causing pancreatitis.

A normal urine analysis and pregnancy test rule out urinary tract infection (UTI) and pregnancy, respectively.

The elevated WBC count indicates infection or inflammation. This is not specific for cholecystitis, as any infection or inflammatory condition can cause inflammation.

The normal AST and ALT, both of which are liver cell enzymes, rule out hepatitis. In acute hepatitis, cellular disruption occurs releasing these enzymes into the circulation. This is important because hepatitis will also present with RUQ pain, as does cholecystitis.

The normal alkaline phosphatase and bilirubin tell us that there are probably no stones in the common duct. Gallstones may move out of the gallbladder and impact in the common duct, blocking the flow of bile. Alkaline phosphatase, which is produced in the common duct cells, elevates in this case as does the bilirubin. In addition, the stool turns light colored since bilirubin is not excreted into the intestines.

The definitive diagnostic test for gallbladder disease is the abdominal ultrasound. The ultrasound demonstrates gallstones (cholelithiasis). However, this by itself doesn't prove the diagnosis of cholecystitis since many people have asymptomatic gallstones. It is when the cystic duct becomes blocked by the stone that symptoms of pain develop (see Fig. 1-4B). If the blockage is complete, the gallbladder distends and the mucous produced by the gallbladder mucosa and bacteria multiply, causing cholecystitis with pain and fever as in this case. The pain is initially visceral in nature and is colicky (comes and goes with gallbladder contraction). As the parietal peritoneum becomes involved with inflammation, the pain becomes constant and is more intense. The complaint of scapula pain is an example of referred pain from the visceral innervation of the gallbladder, which enters the spinal cord with nerves of C3–5, which correspond to the somatic innervation of the skin overlying the scapula. Most patients will improve with fluids and antibiotics. Pain medicine is also given intravenously. Because the recurrence rate of a repeat attack of cholecystitis is very high (>75%), surgery is indicated either on this admission or electively four to six weeks following the acute attack. Once the patient's pain and nausea start to resolve, then fluids are begun by mouth and advanced to solids. The patient is then discharged and scheduled electively for cholecystectomy, or surgery is performed on the same admission. If during the hospitalization the pain and fever progress, then emergency surgery is performed.

DISCUSSION OF MANAGEMENT WITH THE PATIENT

English	Spanish Formal	Spanish Informal
Ms. Martínez, you do have cholecystitis, an inflammation and infection in your gallbladder. This is caused by gallstones causing a blockage in your gallbladder.	Srta. Martínez, usted tiene colecistitis, una inflamación con infección de la vesícula biliar. Esto se debe a cálculos (*piedras*) en la vesícula que bloquean la salida de bilis.	Srta. Martínez, tiene una inflamación de la vesícula causada por piedras que están tapando la salida de la bilis.
Q. Will I need surgery?	¿Voy a necesitar una operación?	¿Me van a operar?
A. In most cases, we recommend surgery to prevent another attack. We will consult a surgeon to evaluate you today.	En la mayoría de los casos, nosotros recomendamos la cirugía para prevenir otro ataque. Hoy mismo vamos a consultar con un cirujano para que evalúe su situación.	Vamos a llamar a un cirujano para que la examine. Por lo general, recomendamos una operación para evitar que tenga otro ataque de dolor.

	English	Spanish Formal	Spanish Informal	Continued
Q.	How long will I be in the hospital?	¿Cuánto tiempo voy a estar en el hospital?	¿Cuánto voy a estar internada?	
A.	That depends. If you continue to improve, you will be here four to five days. Following surgery for this problem, most patients go home the same day or remain in the hospital for one day following surgery. If the surgeon decides to perform surgery, after you are discharged he will schedule that and you will be discharged as soon as you are eating solids and the pain is better.	Eso depende. Si continúa mejorando, va a estar aquí de cuatro a cinco días. La mayoría de los pacientes que son operados de este problema se van para la casa el mismo día o se quedan internados un día más después de la operación. Si el cirujano decide operarla después de que haya salido del hospital, él programará la operación y usted podrá volver a su casa tan pronto como esté comiendo alimentos sólidos y tenga menos dolor.	Depende. Si sigue mejor va a estar aquí cuatro o cinco días. La mayoría de las personas se van para la casa después de la operación o al día siguiente. Si el cirujano decide operarla más adelante, le van a dar la salida cuando esté comiendo comida sólida y tenga menos dolor.	

This is an urgent case of a patient with abdominal pain needing admission to the hospital for treatment and workup. The following case is a more insidious (chronic) presentation of abdominal pain.

CASE 2: COLON CANCER

CHIEF COMPLAINT

A 72-year-old male patient presents with a chief complaint of abdominal pain.

FOCUSED HISTORY

	English	Spanish Formal	Spanish Informal
	Hello Mr. Ramírez, I am George Branton, a third year medical student working with Dr. Gin. I will be asking you some questions and following this I will perform a physical exam.	Hola Señor Ramírez, yo soy George Branton, un estudiante de medicina de tercer año que trabaja con el Dr. Gin. Le voy a hacer algunas preguntas y después un examen físico.	Hola, Señor Ramírez, me llamo George Branton. Soy estudiante de medicina de tercer año. Trabajo con el Dr. Gin. Le voy a hacer unas preguntas y un examen.
Q.	What brings you in to see us today?	¿Por qué vino a vernos el día de hoy?	¿Por qué vino hoy?
A.	I have been having abdominal pain for the last six months.	He estado con dolor de estómago (*panza, vientre, abdomen*) los últimos seis meses.	He tenido dolor de panza desde hace seis meses.
Q.	How old are you?	¿Qué edad tiene?	¿Cuántos años tiene?
A.	Seventy-two years old.	Setenta y dos años de edad.	Setenta y dos.
Q.	Where is the pain located? You can show me.	¿Dónde es el dolor? Muéstreme.	¿Dónde le duele? Enséñeme.
A.	It is hard to describe, it is all over, especially in the lower part of the stomach (patient points to his lower abdomen).	Es difícil describirlo, me duele por todos lados, especialmente en la parte de abajo del estómago (paciente señala el abdomen inferior).	Es difícil decir, es por toda la panza pero más en la parte de abajo.
Q.	How would you describe the pain?	¿Cómo describiría el dolor?	¿Cómo es el dolor?

	English	Spanish Formal	Spanish Informal
A.	It is dull. Like a dull ache. Present all the time.	Es un dolor sordo, como un malestar (*molestia*). Y no se me alivia.	Es como un malestar que no se me quita.
Q.	Is it getting better or worse?	¿Usted diría que el dolor está mejorando o empeorando?	¿Está mejorando o empeorando?
A.	I believe it is getting worse.	Yo creo que está empeorando.	Ahora es peor.
Q.	Have you had associated symptoms such as nausea, vomiting, fever?	¿Ha tenido otros síntomas, como ganas de vomitar (*nausea*), vómito o fiebre?	¿Ha tenido alguna otra cosa, como ganas de vomitar o fiebre?
A.	I feel mildly nauseated after eating and bloated (distended).	Siento un poco de náusea después de comer y como empanzado (*distendido, con el estómago inflamado*).	Tengo ganas de vomitar y me siento empanzado.
Q.	Have you noted a change in your bowel movements, i.e., are they narrower or have you noted blood when you have a bowel movement?	¿Ha notado algún cambio en los excrementos (*las heces, deposiciones*) cuando da del cuerpo (*defeca*), por ejemplo son más delgados o tienen sangre?	¿Ha tenido algún cambio en los excrementos (por ejemplo, con sangre o más delgados)?
A.	My bowel movements have not changed size but I have noted bright red blood on the toilet paper a couple of times following a bowel movement.	Mis heces no han cambiado de tamaño, pero he notado sangre en el papel higiénico un par de veces después de dar del cuerpo (*ir al baño, defecar*).	He visto sangre roja en el papel higiénico un par de veces, pero no ha habido cambios en la forma de los excrementos.
Q.	Have you been more constipated lately or have you had diarrhea?	¿Últimamente ha estado más estreñido (*constipado*) o ha tenido diarrea?	¿Ha estado constipado o tenido diarrea últimamente?
A.	Yes, I have to take a laxative very often to go to the bathroom.	Sí, he tenido que tomar laxantes (*purgantes*) con frecuencia para poder ir al baño.	Sí, he estado tomando purgantes para poder dar del cuerpo.
Q.	Have you lost weight over the past six months?	En los últimos seis meses, ¿ha perdido peso?	¿Ha perdido peso últimamente?
A.	Yes, I have lost about ten pounds.	Sí, he rebajado (*perdido*) como diez libras.	Sí, he bajado como diez libras.
Q.	Have you been more tired lately?	¿Se ha sentido más cansado últimamente?	¿Y se ha sentido cansado?
A.	Yes, I get tired real easily.	Sí, me canso fácilmente.	Sí, ahora me canso con cualquier cosa.
Q.	What makes the pain worse?	¿Qué empeora el dolor?	¿Qué hace peor el dolor?
A.	Eating. After I eat, I get bloated and the pain is more severe. In between eating I feel much better.	Comer. Me siento empanzado (*con el estómago lleno o inflamado*) y me duele más después de comer. Me siento mejor entre las comidas.	Comer. Después de comer me siento empanzado y me duele más el estómago.
Q.	Is the pain constant or does it come and go?	¿El dolor es constante o le va y le viene?	¿Le duele todo el tiempo o le pega y se le quita?
A.	It comes and goes.	Me va y me viene.	Me pega y se me quita.
Q.	Does the pain move or does it stay in the same location?	¿El dolor se mueve o se queda en el mismo lugar?	¿Se mueve para alguna parte?
A.	The pain moves all over the lower stomach.	El dolor se me mueve por toda la parte de abajo del estómago.	Se mueve por la parte de abajo de la panza (*barriga*).
Q.	Do you take any medication for the pain?	¿Toma alguna medicina para el dolor?	¿Toma algo para el dolor?
A.	Just aspirin but it has not helped.	Sólo aspirina pero no me ha ayudado.	Aspirina, pero no sirve para nada.

		English	Spanish Formal	Spanish Informal Continued
Q.		Have you ever had this pain before six months?	¿Ha tenido este dolor alguna vez antes de los últimos seis meses?	¿Ha tenido este dolor antes?
A.		No, that is the first time I noticed it.	No, esa es la primera vez que lo noté (*me pegó*).	No, es la primera vez.
Q.		*Past Medical History*: Have you ever had any gastrointestinal problems before, such as peptic ulcer disease, diverticulitis (inflammation in the colon due to rupture of a diverticulum), appendicitis, gallbladder disease, or hemorrhoids?	*Historia Medica Anterior*: ¿Alguna vez ha tenido otra enfermedad gastrointestinal como úlcera péptica, diverticulitis (inflamación del colon por ruptura de un divertículo), apendicitis, enfermedad de la vesícula biliar o hemorroides?	*Historia Medica Anterior*: ¿Alguna vez ha tenido otra enfermedad del estómago o los intestinos, como úlcera, inflamación del intestino grueso, apendicitis, inflamación de la vesícula o hemorroides?
A.		I had my appendix out when I was a child.	Me sacaron el apéndice cuando era niño (*pequeño*).	Tuve apendicitis cuando era pequeño (*morrito*).
Q.		Do you have a history of heart or lung disease?	¿Ha tenido alguna enfermedad del corazón o los pulmones?	¿Padece del corazón o los pulmones?
A.		No, I am very active and have had no heart or lung problems.	No, yo soy muy activo y nunca he padecido del corazón o de los pulmones.	No, no padezco del corazón ni de los pulmones.
Q.		*Past Surgical History*: Have you ever had surgery besides having your appendix out?	*Historia Quirúrgica Anterior*: Aparte de la operación del apéndice, ¿alguna vez lo han operado?	*Historia Quirúrgica Anterior*: ¿Ha tenido otra operación aparte del apéndice?
A.		I had my tonsils out as a child and had a hernia fixed five years ago.	Me sacaron las amígdalas (*glándulas*) cuando era niño y me operaron de una hernia hace cinco años.	Me operaron de una hernia hace cinco años y de las glándulas cuando era pequeño.
Q.		Have you ever had a colonoscopy or sigmoidoscopy—a test where they put a light in the rectum to see if there is a mass?	¿Alguna vez le han hecho una colonoscopía o una sigmoidoscopía—un examen en el que ponen una luz por el recto para ver si hay un tumor?	¿Alguna vez le han hecho un examen en el que meten un aparato por el recto para ver si hay algún tumor?
A.		About ten years ago they did a sigmoidoscopy which was normal.	Hace como diez años me hicieron una sigmoidoscopía, que resultó normal.	Me hicieron una sigmoidoscopía hace diez años y fue normal.
Q.		*Medications*: What medications do you take?	*Medicamentos*: ¿Qué medicamentos está tomando?	*Medicamentos*: ¿Está tomando alguna medicina?
A.		I take a blood pressure medicine. I can't remember the name.	Tomo una medicina para la presión, pero no me acuerdo del nombre.	Pastillas para la presión, pero no recuerdo el nombre.
Q.		*Social History*: Do you drink alcohol or smoke?	*Historia Social*: ¿Toma alcohol o fuma?	*Historia Social*: ¿Fuma o toma licor?
A.		I smoked up until five years ago and quit. I do not drink.	No tomo licor, pero fumé hasta hace cinco años y lo dejé.	No tomo. Dejé de fumar hace cinco años.
Q.		*Family History*: Is there anyone in your family with a history of cancer, especially colon cancer?	*Historia Familiar*: ¿Alguien en su familia ha padecido de cáncer, especialmente cáncer de colon (*del intestino grueso, de las tripas*)?	*Historia Familiar*: ¿Alguien en su familia ha tenido cáncer?
A.		Not that I know of.	Que yo sepa, no.	No, nadie.

This history is much more in depth than the first case. Here the patient is older and the differential diagnosis is much broader. In the first patient, the pain was localized to the RUQ and she was young, narrowing the differential diagnosis. Here it is diffuse and may be caused by medical as well as surgical causes. With advancing age, the etiology of abdominal pain may include cancer of the intestine (most commonly, colon), diverticular disease of the colon (most commonly, left colon), biliary disease, aortic aneurysm, renal stone, cardiac disease, medications, constipation, etc. (the list is extensive). An ileus (a lack of normal intestinal peristalsis may be caused by certain medications), an infection (urinary or pulmonary), or a metabolic cause such as a low potassium is much more common in elderly patients and may cause abdominal pain. Thus, the history and physical exam is crucial to directing the workup.

FOCUSED PHYSICAL EXAM

The physical exam proceeds as in the above case but is more detailed. It is a complete exam from head to toe, including the rectal exam. An inguinal hernia check is also important in this case. Again, it is crucial to explain to each patient what you are about to do during the physical exam.

English	Spanish Formal	Spanish Informal
Following Abdominal Exam: Mr. Ramírez, I need to perform a rectal exam. I need to check for an inguinal hernia.	Sr. Ramírez, necesito hacerle un tacto rectal (*examen por el recto*). Necesito examinarlo para ver si tiene una hernia inguinal.	Sr. Ramírez, necesito hacerle un examen por el recto y examinarlo para ver si tiene una hernia inguinal.

PERTINENT PHYSICAL FINDINGS

The abdomen is mildly distended and tympanitic to percussion. Bowel sounds are normal. There is minimal tenderness to deep palpation in all quadrants. No voluntary or involuntary guarding is present. Rectal exam reveals a prolapsing internal hemorrhoid, no masses are palpated, and the prostate is smooth and mildly enlarged. No gross blood is present, but the stool is guiac positive (occult blood is present).

DIFFERENTIAL DIAGNOSIS

The importance of this list cannot be stressed enough. It is based on your history and physical exam. It allows one to proceed logically in the patient's workup. Without it, the workup would go forward without direction, in a random manner. Most of us Attendings believe this list most accurately reflects a student's thought process.

English	Spanish Formal	Spanish Informal
• Partial large bowel obstruction (secondary to colon cancer) • Partial small bowel obstruction	• Obstrucción parcial del intestino grueso (secundaria a cáncer del colon) • Obstrucción parcial del intestino delgado	• Obstrucción del intestino grueso • Obstrucción del intestino delgado • Íleo

English	Spanish Formal	Spanish Informal Continued
• Ileus (non-mechanical obstruction) • Hemorrhoids	• Íleo (obstrucción no mecánica) • Hemorroides	• Hemorroides
Mr. Ramírez, I am concerned about some of the findings on history and physical exam. Bloating, abdominal pain after eating and weight loss may be a sign of partial obstruction due to scar tissue from your prior surgery or a blockage in the colon. The bleeding may be due to internal hemorrhoids. However, the presence of symptoms such as these makes us want to be sure that it is not from a colon cancer. We will order some blood tests and x-rays of your stomach to see if there is a partial blockage. We will see you back in clinic after these tests are done.	Sr. Ramírez, estoy preocupado por algunos hallazgos de la historia y el examen físico. Sentirse empanzado (*lleno*) y con dolor abdominal después de comer, y perder peso pueden ser signos de una obstrucción parcial del intestino. Esto se puede deber a cicatrices (*tejido de cicatrización*) de la operación anterior o a una obstrucción del colon. El sangrado se puede deber a hemorroides internas. Sin embargo, la presencia de estos síntomas nos llevan a querer estar seguros (*descartar*) de que no hay un cáncer de colon. Le vamos a hacer unos exámenes de sangre y radiografías del estómago para ver si hay una obstrucción parcial del intestino. Lo veremos nuevamente en la clínica después de que le hayan hecho estos exámenes.	Estoy preocupada por sus síntomas. Tener dolor de panza después de comer, sentirse empanzado y perder peso pueden ser síntomas de una obstrucción del intestino por las cicatrices de la operación anterior o de un bloqueo del intestino grueso. El sangrado puede ser por hemorroides internas. Pero de todas maneras, para estar seguros, es mejor hacerle otros exámenes para descartar un cáncer del colon. Le voy a mandar unos exámenes de sangre y unas radiografías del estómago. Lo quiero volver a ver una vez que tenga los resultados.
(It is very important when one is suspicious of cancer that the patient also be told of the possible benign conditions that can cause the same symptoms.)	(Cuando un médico sospecha que su paciente tiene cáncer, es muy importante conversar con él sobre otros padecimientos benignos que pueden causar los mismos síntomas).	

Does the patient need to be admitted to the hospital for the workup, as was the case for the first patient?

If you said no, you were right. He is holding down food, he has no infection that needs to be treated; there is no guarding on abdominal exam. It is not an acute event, i.e., it has been going on for the past six months. This patient can be worked up as an outpatient.

What ancillary tests do you want to order (start with simplest, least invasive tests)?

A complete blood count (CBC) will tell us if the patient is anemic from chronic blood loss, as may happen with colon cancer.

Radiographs of the abdomen will show us the gas pattern of the intestine and may help differentiate ileus and colon obstruction from small bowel obstruction (Figs. 1-5, 1-6, and 1-7).

Ultimately, this patient will need a colonoscopy due to his age, blood per rectum, and obstructive symptoms to rule out colon cancer. Most obstructing colon cancers involve the left colon due to the nature of the formed stool and the fact that cancers on the left side grow circumferentially. Cancer of the right colon presents with anemia due to occult blood loss (the blood is mixed

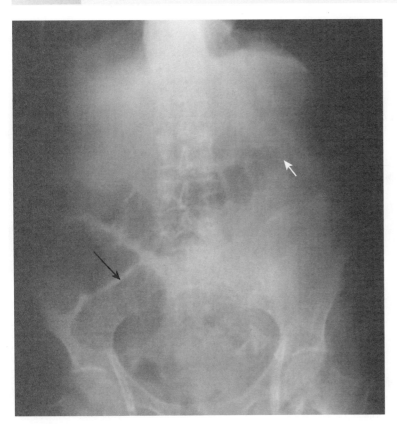

Figure 1-5. Abdominal radiographs demonstrating dilated right colon in a patient with colon cancer. Note the dilated cecum (*white arrow*) and the "cutoff" (*black arrow*) indicating an obstructing lesion.

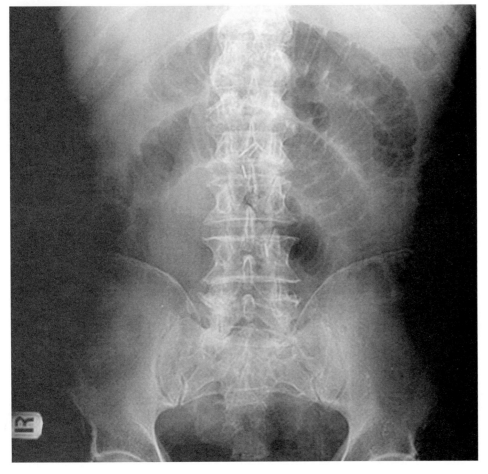

Figure 1-6. Small bowel obstruction from adhesions. Abdominal radiograph. Note the dilated small bowel (central location) and the appearance of the plica semilunaris appearing as "stacked coins" (*arrow*).

Figure 1-7. A patient with an ileus (non-mechanical obstruction) resulting from hypokalemia. Abdominal radiograph. Note the dilated transverse colon signified by haustra (*arrow*).

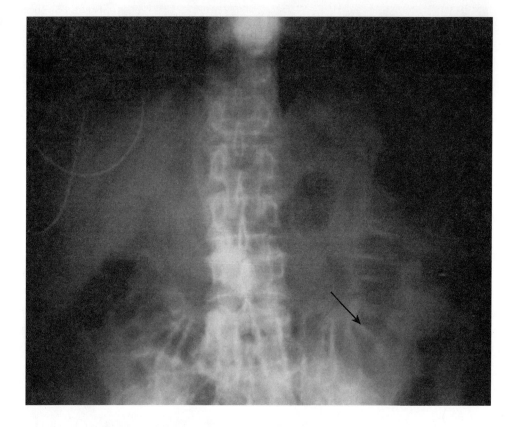

in with the stool so as to not be noticed by the patient). Obstruction is uncommon on the right side of the colon due to the liquid nature of the stool on the right side. The bleeding from left-sided colon cancers is bright red. Although bright red blood per rectum is often caused by internal hemorrhoids, colon cancer needs to be excluded.

TEST RESULTS

- WBC Hemoglobin/Hematocrit: 14.2/45.2
- Abdominal radiographs: (see Fig. 1-5, large bowel gas with cutoff sign [*arrow*])
- Colonoscopy: (Fig. 1-8)
- Biopsy results: Infiltrating adenocarcinoma

Many colon cancers are curable depending upon the stage of disease. This is determined following resection of the part of the colon that is involved with the tumor (in this case, the sigmoid colon). Prognosis and further treatment such as chemotherapy will depend on the depth of tumor involvement of the colon wall, whether adjacent lymph nodes are involved with tumor and whether there is tumor metastasis. This is determined by the pathologist after the colon is removed surgically. Note that the patient is not anemic (hemoglobin and hematocrit are normal). Right-sided colon cancer presents most commonly with anemia, while left-sided tumors present with obstruction and bright red blood per rectum. Although rectal bleeding is commonly caused by hemorrhoids (as is illustrated by this case), in any patient over the age of 50 with rectal bleeding, left-sided colon cancer has to be ruled out by endoscopy.

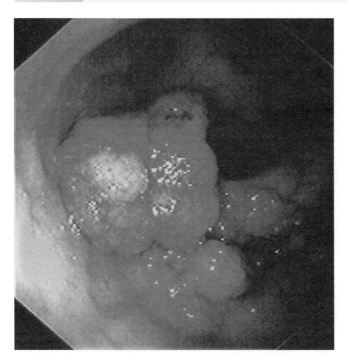

Figure 1-8. Colonoscopy demonstrating a mass in the colon. (From Townsend C: *Sabiston Textbook of Surgery*, ed 17, Philadelphia, Saunders, 2004.)

DISCUSSION OF MANAGEMENT WITH THE PATIENT

	English	Spanish Formal	Spanish Informal
	The doctor returns: Mr. Ramírez, we have all the results of your tests. Your abdominal problems of pain, constipation, and bleeding are due to a partial blockage of the colon by a tumor. The biopsy they did shows a colon cancer. The usual treatment is surgery to remove the cancer and the part of the colon that is involved. I have made an appointment with a surgeon to discuss this option with you. I know you must have many questions and I will try to answer them.	*El doctor regresa*: Sr. Ramírez, tenemos todos los resultados de los exámenes. Los problemas abdominales de dolor, estreñimiento y sangrado se deben a un bloqueo parcial del colon por un tumor. La biopsia que le hicieron muestra que es un cáncer de colon. El tratamiento usual es cirugía para quitar (*remover*) el cáncer y la parte del colon que está afectada (*comprometida*). Ya le hice una cita con un cirujano para que hable con usted sobre esta opción. Yo sé que usted debe de tener muchas preguntas y las voy a tratar de contestar.	*El médico regresa*: Sr. Ramírez, los resultados de los exámenes demuestran que usted tiene una obstrucción del intestino grueso por un tumor. Y la biopsia nos dice que es un cáncer del colon. Generalmente, el tratamiento es una operación para quitar el cáncer y la parte del intestino afectada. Le hice una cita con un cirujano para que converse con usted sobre las opciones que tiene en este momento. ¿Tiene preguntas?
Q.	What exactly does the surgery consist of?	Específicamente, ¿en qué consiste la operación?	¿Cómo es la operación?
A.	I am not a surgeon, and he or she will discuss this in much greater detail as to the exact procedure and risks. The surgery is done in the operating room with you asleep, called general anesthesia. They then open the stomach and remove the diseased part of the colon, following which they sew the two ends of the colon	Yo no soy cirujano y él/ella le explicará con más detalle en qué consiste la operación y cuáles son los riesgos. La cirugía se realiza en una sala de operaciones con usted dormido, bajo anestesia general. Los cirujanos abren el estómago y quitan la parte enferma del colon. Luego cosen los dos extremos del colon para unirlos y cierran el estómago nuevamente.	No soy cirujano y él o ella le va a explicar mejor los detalles de la operación, pero le puedo decir que la cirugía se hace en el hospital. Lo van a dormir con anestesia general. El cirujano le va a abrir la panza para quitar el tumor y la parte enferma del intestino. Después van a coser los dos cabos que quedan para pegarlos y cerrar

	English	Spanish Formal	Spanish Informal Continued
	together and close the stomach. You will get strong pain medicines after surgery and remain in the hospital for about a week until the colon starts working and you are eating.	Después de la operación, le van a dar medicinas fuertes para el dolor. Se va a quedar internado en el hospital por una semana hasta que el colon comience a funcionar y usted esté comiendo otra vez.	la panza otra vez. Después le van a dar medicinas para el dolor y se va quedar internado hasta que comience a sanar y esté comiendo bien.
Q.	What are my chances of not making it?	¿Qué posibilidades hay de que no sobreviva a la operación?	¿Me puedo morir en la operación?
A.	This is a serious problem, but many people are alive and well following treatment for colon cancer. The surgeon will discuss the risks of the surgery, but in general, patients do very well after this type of surgery. It is normal to associate death with cancer, but many people are cured by surgery and are alive today.	Este es un problema serio, pero muchas personas sobreviven y continúan con sus vidas después del tratamiento de cáncer de colon. El cirujano conversará con usted sobre los riesgos de esta cirugía, pero en general, a los pacientes les va muy bien después de este tipo de operación. Es normal que las personas asocien el cáncer con la muerte, pero muchas personas se han curado con la operación y ahora están disfrutando de la vida.	El cirujano le va a decir más sobre los riesgos de la operación, pero a la mayoría de las personas les va muy bien y continúan con sus vidas después de la cirugía. Es normal que cuando la persona oye la palabra "cáncer" piense en la muerte, pero muchas personas se curan con la operación y siguen viviendo bastante bien.

It is of utmost importance to address the fears of a patient following giving them the news of cancer. Most nonmedical people associate cancer with pain, suffering, and ultimate death. Although specifics of the surgery are left to the surgeon, the primary care doctor should have a general idea about the surgery.

CASE 3: APPENDICITIS

The first patient represents an urgent (case-1) case, where hospitalization is required but emergency surgery is not. The second patient represents a case where the disease process is chronic and although serious, does not require admission to the hospital for workup. What remains is the presentation of a patient with a disease process that requires hospitalization and emergent surgery for a potentially life-threatening problem. Bleeding or hemorrhage with hemodynamic instability is one example. An instance of this is a ruptured aortic aneurysm. The clinical presentation is abdominal and back pain, shock, and a pulsatile abdominal mass (the ruptured aneurysm) (Fig. 1-9). Survival is inversely correlated with delay in surgical intervention. The other indication for emergency surgery is for peritonitis. This includes perforated bowel with accompanying peritonitis such as a perforated duodenal ulcer, ruptured colonic diverticulum with peritonitis, and acute appendicitis.

CHIEF COMPLAINT

A 15-year-old male patient presents with right-sided abdominal pain. (Again, because of the young age of the patient and the more limited possibilities, a more focused history and physical exam are performed.)

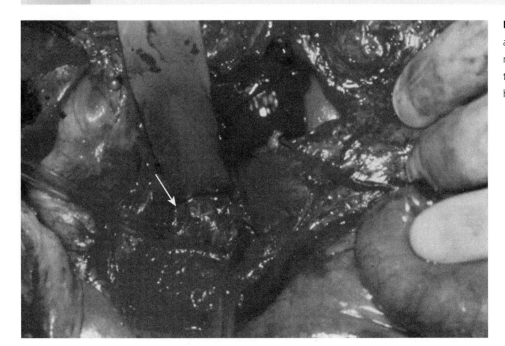

Figure 1-9. Ruptured abdominal aortic aneurysm. Note the large retroperitoneal hematoma due to containment of the hemorrhage (*arrow*).

HISTORY

	English	Spanish Formal	Spanish Informal
Q.	How are you, Bobby? I am Dr. Smith and I am going to ask you some questions, okay?	¿Cómo está, Bobby? Soy la Dra. Smith y le voy a hacer unas preguntas. ¿Está bien?	Hola, Bobby. ¿Cómo está? Soy la Dra. Smith y le voy a hacer unas preguntas. ¿Está bien?
A.	Yes, that is okay.	Sí, está bien.	Sí.
Q.	How old are you?	¿Qué edad tiene?	¿Cuántos años tiene?
A.	I will be sixteen in two weeks.	Voy a cumplir dieciseis en dos semanas.	Casi dieciseis.
Q.	What brings you here today?	¿Por qué vino hoy?	¿Por qué razón vino hoy?
A.	I have real bad stomach pains.	Tengo mucho dolor de estómago.	Tengo bastante dolor de estómago.
Q.	When did the pain begin?	¿Cuándo le comenzó el dolor?	¿Desde cuándo le duele?
A.	It began yesterday.	Me comenzó ayer.	Desde ayer.
Q.	Where did the pain begin? Has it changed or moved?	¿Dónde le comenzó el dolor? ¿Ha cambiado, o se le ha movido?	¿Dónde le comenzó? ¿Se le ha movido?
A.	It began around my belly button and the upper center part of my stomach	Me comenzó por el ombligo y la parte de arriba del centro del estómago.	Comenzó por el ombligo y el centro del estómago.
Q.	Has it changed or moved?	¿Ha cambiado o se ha movido?	¿Se ha movido?
A.	Today it is on the lower right side.	Me comenzó alrededor del ombligo, pero hoy está en el lado derecho, aquí abajo (*cuadrante inferior derecho*).	Pues me comenzó por el ombligo pero ahora lo tengo en el lado derecho, aquí abajo.
Q.	Have you had diarrhea or constipation?	¿Ha tenido diarrea o estreñimiento?	¿Ha estado constipado o flojo del estómago?
A.	I haven't had diarrhea or constipation.	No he tenido diarrea ni estreñimiento.	No he tenido diarrea ni he estado constipado.

	English	Spanish Formal	Spanish Informal Continued
Q.	Have you had nausea or vomiting?	¿Ha tenido náusea o vómito?	¿Ha tenido ganas de vomitar?
A.	Today I have had nausea and vomited once.	Hoy he tenido ganas de vomitar y vomité una vez.	Sí, hoy vomité una vez.
Q.	Have you had fever or chills?	¿Ha tenido fiebre o escalofríos?	¿Ha tenido calentura o escalofríos?
A.	I feel warm today but haven't taken my temperature.	Me siento afiebrado hoy pero no me he tomado la temperatura.	Me siento caliente pero no me he tomado la temperatura.
Q.	Have you had this pain before?	¿Ha tenido este dolor anteriormente?	¿Ha tenido este dolor antes?
A.	No, I haven't had pain like this before.	No, nunca he tenido un dolor como este.	No.
Q.	Have you had any cough or sore throat?	¿Ha tenido tos o infección en la garganta?	¿Ha tenido tos o dolor de garganta?
A.	No, not recently.	No, no me ha dado últimamente.	No.
Q.	Have you lost your appetite?	¿Ha perdido el apetito (*las ganas de comer*)?	¿Tiene apetito?
A.	Yes, today I am not hungry.	Sí, hoy no tengo hambre.	Hoy estoy sin hambre.
Q.	Did it hurt on the car ride here? Does it hurt to walk?	¿Le dolió en el automóvil cuando venía para acá? ¿Le duele cuando camina?	¿Le dolía cuando venía en el auto (*carro, coche*) o le duele cuando camina?
A.	Yes, when I move it is really painful.	Sí, cuando me muevo me duele mucho.	Sí, me duele más cuando me muevo.

PHYSICAL EXAM – PERTINENT FINDINGS

Abdominal exam: Involuntary guarding and rebound is noted in the RLQ.

What is rebound?

When you push on the abdomen gently and then release, the patient has more pain upon release. This sudden movement of the abdominal wall and underlying viscera causes this sudden pain with release. This is a sign of peritonitis (inflammation of the parietal peritoneum).

DIFFERENTIAL DIAGNOSIS

Remember your anatomy! Right lower quadrant pain in a young man—there are limited possibilities.

English	Spanish Formal	Spanish Informal
• Appendicitis	• Apendicitis	• Apendicitis
• Mesenteric adenitis	• Adenitis mesentérica	• Adenitis mesentérica
• Crohn's disease	• Enfermedad de Crohn	• Enfermedad de Crohn
• Meckel's diverticulitis	• Diverticulitis de Meckels	• Diverticulitis de Meckels
• Abdominal pain etiology unknown	• Dolor abdominal de etiología desconocida	• Dolor abdominal de origen desconocido

Lower abdominal pain in a young man: Always list appendicitis, especially if it is right-sided.

Mesenteric adenitis: This is often confused with appendicitis. In the terminal ileum (located in the right lower quadrant) there is a rich supply of lymph nodes in the mesentery. Following a viral upper respiratory infection or after Strep throat, these lymph nodes enlarge and stretch the mesentery, causing RLQ pain. Although pain is present, anorexia is less often present as it is in appendicitis.

Crohn's disease: Also termed inflammatory bowel disease (IBD), this disorder most often involves the terminal ileum. This disease is an autoimmune disease that can affect the gastrointestinal tract from the mouth to the anus, but most often affects the terminal ileum and next often the colon. Right lower quadrant pain may be the initial presentation of IBD. Clinical symptoms—including diarrhea, pain, and weight loss due to malabsorption—are usually also present.

Inguinal hernia: May present at any age with lower abdominal pain, especially if intestine is incarcerated (trapped) in the hernia sac (Fig. 1-10).

Meckel's diverticulitis: Can present with RLQ pain. Meckel's diverticulum is found in the terminal ileum within two feet of the ileo-cecal valve. Half of these diverticula will contain gastric mucosa, thus perforation may occur. It is much more common in the pediatric population.

Finally, many things in medicine do not have a scientific explanation. Clinically we see patients with abdominal pain, including right-sided abdominal pain, who get better without a definitive diagnosis or treatment.

Before deciding what labs or X-rays we want, based on the above history and physical findings, is this elective? Can we send the patient home and work him up as an outpatient, do we need to admit the patient to the hospital for observation and possible surgery, or should the patient undergo surgery as soon as possible?

This patient clearly can't be discharged home. He has nausea and vomiting, fever, involuntary guarding, and rebound (signs of peritonitis). Movement causes the pain to worsen (e.g., the car ride to the hospital). These patients classically bend over to walk due to the peritonitis and lay very still. He needs surgery as soon as possible. The next step is to place an intravenous catheter to give fluids intravenously. As noted above, due to the vomiting and intra-abdominal inflammation, most such patients are moderately dehydrated. The administration of intravenous normal saline or Ringer's Lactate will allow stabilization of the intravascular volume. This in turn will allow the surgery to proceed much more smoothly.

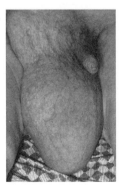

Figure 1-10. Large inguinal hernia in an elderly patient. Note swelling in the scrotum due to loops of bowel in the scrotal sac.

Next, a CBC is usually ordered. Typically, in appendicitis, the WBC is elevated, but this is not 100%. Thus, appendicitis is a clinical diagnosis.

DISCUSSION OF MANAGEMENT WITH THE PATIENT

	English	Spanish Formal	Spanish Informal
	(Talking to Bobby's mother as well as Bobby): Based on your history and physical exam, I believe we need to remove your appendix. We can't be 100% sure that is what it is, but to delay may allow the appendix to rupture.	(Hablando con la mamá de Bobby y con Bobby): De acuerdo con la historia y el examen físico, yo pienso que debemos operarlo para removerle el apéndice. No podemos estar ciento por ciento seguros de que es eso, pero si esperamos, el apéndice se puede romper.	(Conversando con Bobby y su mamá): Yo pienso que Bobby tiene apendicitis, así que vamos a tener que operarlo para quitarle el apéndice. No podemos estar ciento por ciento seguros, pero si esperamos, el apéndice puede explotar.
Q.	How long will I be in the hospital?	¿Cuánto tiempo voy a estar en el hospital?	¿Cuánto voy a estar internado?
A.	You will be in the hospital about one to two days. When you can eat we will send you home.	Va a estar en el hospital como uno o dos días. Cuando pueda comer, le daremos la salida.	Va a estar internado unos dos días. Cuando esté comiendo otra vez, le damos la salida.
Q.	Will it hurt after the surgery?	¿Me va a doler después de la operación?	¿Voy a tener dolor después de la operación?
A.	Yes, but we will give you strong medicines for the pain.	Sí, pero le vamos a dar medicinas fuertes para el dolor.	Sí, pero le vamos a dar medicinas para el dolor.
Q.	When can I go back to school?	¿Cuándo voy a poder regresar a la escuela?	¿Cuándo voy a poder volver a la escuela?
A.	Usually in about one week you can return to school. Generally, you need to wait about six weeks before competitive sports are started.	Generalmente, las personas pueden regresar a la escuela en una semana. Y tienen que esperar seis semanas antes de participar en deportes competitivos.	Como una semana después de la operación, pero tiene que esperar unas seis semanas para participar en deportes.

Following rapid resuscitation with intravenous fluids (1 to 2 liters), the patient is taken to surgery for appendectomy. We always tell the patient that there is a chance that the appendix will be normal and that some other pathology might be found (see differential diagnosis).

A NOTE ON APPENDICITIS

Classically in appendicitis, the pain begins in the peri-umbilical region. Initially, the disease begins as an obstruction of the appendix by a fecalith or, more commonly, hypertrophy of the lymphatics in the appendix. Distally, mucous continues to be secreted into the lumen of the appendix, causing distention (visceral pain) referred to the peri-umbilical region. As the disease progresses, the serosa of the appendix becomes inflamed (Fig. 1-11), as does the parietal peritoneum of the abdominal wall producing right lower quadrant pain and involuntary guarding. This process takes between 12 and 24 hours. Early in the disease, anorexia is noted. Fever takes a little longer to develop and when it occurs is low grade, i.e., 38° C.

Often the diagnosis is not as clear as the above case, and then a number of options exist. If we suspect appendicitis but the diagnosis is unclear, we admit

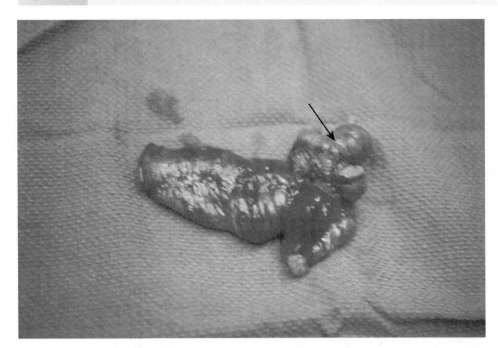

Figure 1-11. Gross pathology of a removed appendix in a 16-year-old male patient with clinical symptoms of appendicitis. Note arrow demonstrating perforation of the appendiceal tip.

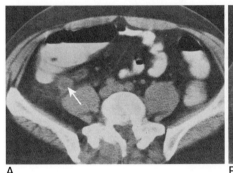

A

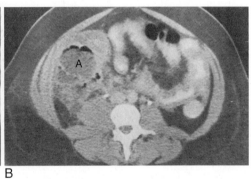

B

Figure 1-12. CT scan demonstrating appendicitis. (From Townsend C: *Sabiston Textbook of Surgery*, ed 17, Philadelphia, Saunders, 2004.)

the patient to the hospital and may order a computed tomography (CT) scan, which might demonstrate appendiceal wall thickening (Fig. 1-12). In the female patient, ovarian and fallopian tube diseases can present with symptoms similar to appendicitis. (This will be discussed in Chapter 4.) In this group of patients, ancillary tests such as CT and ultrasound are often used. In the above patient, where the symptoms are classic, no tests are necessary.

VOCABULARY

English	Español
Abdomen	Estómago, abdomen, panza, barriga
Abdominal cramps	Cólicos, retortijones, cólicos abdominales, punzadas
Abdominal pain	Dolor de panza, dolor de estómago, dolor de barriga, dolor de tripa, dolor abdominal

English	Español	Continued
Admit into the hospital	Internarlo(a) en el hospital, ingresarlo(a) en el hospital	
Ancillary tests	Exámenes auxiliares, complementarios, pruebas de laboratorio	
Anemia	Anemia, falta de hierro	
Aortic aneurysm	Aneurisma de la aorta	
Appendectomy	Apendicectomía, operación de la apéndice	
Belly button	Ombligo	
Bloated, distended	Distendido, empanzado, hinchado, inflamado, lleno de aire	
Blood pressure	Presión arterial, presión de la sangre, la presión	
Bowel movement	Dar del cuerpo, defecar, obrar, deposición, evacuar el vientre	
Bowel obstruction	Obstrucción intestinal, obstrucción de los intestinos, las tripas	
Bowel sounds	Ruidos peristálticos, ruidos intestinales, borborigmos	
Burning pain	Dolor quemante, "... como que me queman con fuego", ardor	
Chemotherapy	Quimioterapia, tratamiento para el cáncer	
Cholelithiasis	Colelitiasis, inflamación de la vesícula por cálculos o piedras que obstruyen el paso de bilis	
Colon cancer	Cáncer de colon, cáncer del intestino grueso	
Colonic diverticulum	Divertículo del colon	
Colonoscopy	Colonoscopía, examen de los intestinos	
Constant pain	Dolor constante, dolor todo el tiempo, dolor cansado	
Constipated	Constipado, estreñido, apretado, con dificultad para dar del cuerpo	
Dull pain	Dolor sordo, dolor lerdo, "... como una molestia"	
Elective surgery	Cirugía electiva, operación que se puede programar con tiempo	
Fecalith	Fecalito, excremento pequeño	
Feces	Excrementos, heces, materia fecal	
Gallbladder	Vesícula biliar, la vesícula, la bilis	
Gallstones	Piedras en la vesícula, Cálculos biliares	
Gastrointestinal tract	Tracto gastrointestinal, aparato gastrointestinal	
Hematocrit	Hematocrito, el porcentaje de glóbulos rojos en una muestra de sangre	
Hemoglobin	Hemoglobina, proteína que contiene hierro y que se encuentra dentro de los glóbulos rojos de la sangre	
Hypertrophy	Hipertrofia, crecimiento de las células de un músculo	
Incarcerated	Encarcerada, estrangulada	
Inflammatory bowel disease	Enfermedad Inflamatoria del Intestino	

English	Español
Inguinal hernia	Hernia inguinal, hernia
Intravenous fluid	Suero intravenoso, suero por la vena
Large intestine	Intestino grueso, mondongo
Liver cirrhosis	Cirrosis hepática, cirrosis del hígado
Lose weight	Perder peso, perder libras, bajar de peso, rebajar de peso
Lymph nodes	Nódulos linfáticos, ganglios linfáticos
Myocardial infarction	Infarto del miocardio, ataque del corazón, infarto
Nausea	Náusea, ganas de vomitar, basca
Occult blood	Sangre oculta
Outpatient clinic	Clínica de consulta externa, consulta externa
Pathologist	Patólogo, especialista en patología
Pelvic exam	Examen pélvico, examen vaginal, examen ginecológico
Perforated bowel	Intestino perforado
Perforated duodenal ulcer	Úlcera duodenal perforada
Peritonitis	Peritonitis, inflamación del peritoneo
Prolapsing internal hemorrhoid	Hemorroide interna prolapsada
Rebound	Rebote
Rectal bleeding	Sangrado rectal, sangrado por el recto, sangre en los excrementos
Rectal exam	Examen rectal, tacto rectal
Renal stone	Piedra del riñón, cálculo renal, urolitiasis
Scar tissue	Cicatriz, tejido de cicatrización
Sharp pain	Dolor agudo, dolor punzante, dolor lacerante
Sigmoid colon	Colon sigmoides
Small intestine	Intestino delgado, tripas
Stool guiac test	Prueba de guayaco en los excrementos (las heces)
Strep throat	Infección de la garganta, faringitis estreptocócica, infección de la garganta por estreptococos
Tachycardia	Taquicardia
"... the pain hits me after eating"	"... el dolor me pega (o comienza) después de comer"
Throbbing pain	Dolor punzante, "... como una puñalada". Dolor pulsátil o pulsante.
To have diarrhea	Tener diarrea, andar mal del estómago, andar flojo
Urinary tract infection	Infección de las vías urinarias, infección de orina, mal de orín

GRAMMATICAL TIPS

Certain verbs repeat themselves during the History and Physical Exam of a patient. We will concentrate on these during this and subsequent chapters. Particular attention will be given to the present, past (preterite and imperfect forms), and past perfect tense of these verbs.

REVIEW OF THE PRESENT TENSE

To conjugate a verb, the endings are taken off and the root or stem of the verb is left by itself.

Example: *Hablar – Comer – Vivir:* the endings *-ar, -er,* and *-ir* are dropped leaving *habl-, com-,* and *viv-* as the stems. Then, to conjugate you have to add the endings depending on the subject: I, you, he, etc.

For the present tense, the endings are as follows:

Verb Subject	*Hablar* = to speak	*Comer* = to eat	*Vivir* = to live
I = *Yo*	Habl – **o**	Com – **o**	Viv – **o**
You (informal) = *Tú*	Habl – **as**	Com – **es**	Viv – **es**
He/She/You (formal) = *El/Ella/Usted*	Habl – **a**	Com – **e**	Viv – **e**
We = *Nosotros, Nosotras*	Habl – **amos**	Com – **emos**	Viv – **imos**
You (plural)/They = *Ustedes, Ellos, Ellas*	Habl – **an**	Com – **en**	Viv – **en**

Stem-changing Verbs

There are verbs that are stem-changing, which means that a vowel in the stem of the verb will change. The only form that does not change is the nosotros (we). In the case where there is more than one vowel, the second vowel is the one that is changed. The four stem changes are: o-ue, e-i, e-ie, and u-ue. This also means that the verb that does not have the stem-changing vowels will not be stem-changing at all.

The following verbs are stem-changing. Pay close attention to the stem and how it changes.

Dormir = to sleep	*Repetir* = to repeat	*Preferir* = to prefer	*Jugar* = to play
Duermo	Repito	Prefiero	Juego
Duermes	Repites	Prefieres	Juegas
Duerme	Repite	Prefiere	Juega
Dormimos	Repetimos	Preferimos	Jugamos
Duermen	Repiten	Prefieren	Juegan

Spelling Changes

Spelling changes occur in the verbs that have an unstressed I in between two vowels. This is a phonetics rule. In many cases, phonetics rules over grammar in the Spanish language. For example, the verb construir in the "yo" form changes its spelling to construyo.

The following verbs are some examples of the verbs that have spelling changes in the *"yo"* form.

To say = Decir = digo

To do or make = hacer = hago

To have = tener = tengo

To know = conocer = conozco

To drive = conducir = conduzco

To obtain = conseguir = consigo

Then, there are the irregular verbs that do not follow any rules and have different stems and endings. Some examples are: *ser, estar, ir,* etc.

EXERCISE 1

Fill in the blanks with the correct conjugation of the verb in the present indicative tense:

Los mamografias _____ (*ser*) importantes para detectar la existencia de tumores malignos y beningnos.

Los doctores _____ (*examinar*) a los pacientes en el consultorio.

El cáncer del seno _____ (*ser*) una causa de muerte de las mujeres en los Estados Unidos.

Los médicos _____ (*decir*) que la prevención del cáncer _____ (*tener*) sus bases en la regularidad de las mujeres para hacerse mamografias regularmente.

EXERCISE 2

Conjugate the following verbs in the present tense: Salir, tener(ie), conseguir(i), tomar, mover(ue), estar

Tener: To Have
This is the verb most commonly used in the History and Physical Exam. *Tener* is a *"yo"* irregular verb as well as a stem-changing verb. It means "to have" or "to possess." Thus, it is used to describe many symptoms of disease states, for example:

"*¿Tiene dolor?*" = Do you have pain?

Simple present:

Yo tengo = I have	*Nosotros, nosotras tenemos* = We have
Tú tienes = You have	*Ustedes tienen* = You all have
Ella, él, usted* tiene = He or she has	*Ellos, ellas tienen* = They have

* *Usted* is a subject pronoun and it means *you* in a formal setting. It is used when addressing adults or strangers in formal situations, for example: "*Usted tiene apendicitis*" = "You have appendicitis." This expression is used only when you meet people for the first time and you are not acquainted with them.

Commands in the present are formed using the third person singular, "*él*" or "*ella*" form for *tú* commands. They also change the ending of the "*yo*" in the present to an *-e* for *-ar*-ending verbs and use an *-a* for *-er* and *-ir* verbs to form commands in the "*usted*" form. For example, *hablar* becomes *habla* for "*tú*" and *hable* for "*usted.*"

EXERCISE 3

Practice by changing the following verbs in the command form: Comer, vestir(i), ir (irreg.), levantar, sentar(ie), poner.

REFLEXIVE VERBS AND THEIR PRONOUNS

These types of verbs are characterized by the *-se* endings, which means these are things one does to oneself. For example, "*me levanto*" means "I wake up myself."

The reflexive pronouns are *me* (myself), *te* (yourself), *se* (himself, herself, yourself; formal, yourselves and themselves) and *nos* (ourselves). When constructing a command, the reflexive pronoun is attached to the verb (*dime dónde te duele*).

Doler: To Hurt

The verb *doler* means "to hurt." During the history and physical exam, we commonly use the third person *duele* or *duelen* (plural) because of the structure of verbs like *doler* and *gustar*. When using these types of verbs, the part that hurts is the subject. When using these verbs, do not translate literally. So if you use the verb *doler*, then it is a part (or parts) of the body that hurts. For example, "*Me duele el estómago*" is literally translated as "*The stomach hurts me.*" The stomach is the subject of this sentence and I am the object. Therefore, if what is hurting is the legs, then you use the plural form, which is *duelen*.

In conversation, people often use the indirect object pronouns *me, te,* or *le* accompanying the verb *doler*. For example:

> "*¿Qué le duele?*" = What hurts you (him, her)?
> "*Me duele antes de comer*" = It hurts before eating.
> "*¿Te duele el estómago?*" = Does your stomach hurt?

Notice that in each case the pronoun *me, te,* or *le* is placed before the verb *doler*. Indirect objects receive the action of the verb indirectly and the pronouns indicate to whom or for whom an action is done. In the above example, *le* represents "you" (formal), but it also could represent "him" or "her" in a phrase like "*¿Qué le duele?*" That *le* is very ambiguous, and to clarify the person you must add a prepositional phrase: *a Pedro* or *a Sonia* will clarify that *le* is either *Pedro* (him) or *Sonia* (her).

When the subject (what hurts) is plural, the verb *doler* also becomes plural by adding an "*n*." For example,

"Me duele la pierna" = My leg hurts (The leg is hurting me)
"Me duelen las piernas" = My legs hurt (The legs are hurting me)

Keep in mind that these verbs use a different structure and you will only use the singular or plural form of the third person.

CULTURAL TIPS: THE LATINO FAMILY

Culture plays an important role in the way patients think and decide on issues related to health and disease. In this and the following chapters, we will examine some cultural values, beliefs, and practices that should be taken into account when caring for Latino patients.

The *familia* is very important for Latino patients, as for other cultures. The typical Latino family includes extended family members, such as grandparents, aunts, uncles, cousins, in-laws and even *padrinos* (godparents) and neighbors. The family is a social and support system that is essential to the development of societies in the world—therefore, the typical Latin American family includes many members and negotiates decisions that will affect the family in general.

Latino patients have a strong tendency to consult health-related decisions with family members. In some cases—especially patients with serious medical conditions—the family basically assumes the responsibility to watch over, care for, and sometimes even "think" for the sick member. The justification for this protective attitude seems to be that Latino families believe that the sick person should concentrate all his or her energy and strength in fighting the disease while they "think" about the healing strategy and take care of his/her immediate needs. At the same time, the family believes that support is shown at these situations where your true friends and family are there, active and ready to help with any needs that might present.

Health professionals taking care of Latino patients should be aware of this cultural value and make efforts to communicate with family members about the patient's condition without violating his or her right to confidentiality.

2 Chest Pain

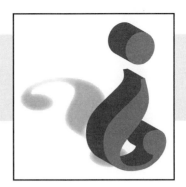

INTRODUCTION

Chest pain is a commonly encountered symptom in emergency departments as well as outpatient clinics. There are many etiologies that cause chest pain that range from life-threatening diseases to minor illness. The key to handling a patient with chest pain is to assess whether the pain is of cardiac or noncardiac origin. Pain of cardiac origin is a red flag, often indicating a serious underlying condition. To determine the origin of chest pain, one must rely on the initial evaluation, your observations, or "eye balling" the patient as we say in medicine. This is a critical first step in evaluating all patients with chest pain as well as other illnesses such as abdominal pain. Someone with a serious clinical problem such as a myocardial infarction (MI) will be agitated, sweating, often in acute distress. A patient with a pulmonary embolus will be breathing rapidly due to the hypoxemia caused by the embolus to the lung. Next, history, physical exam, and finally lab tests will confirm your clinical suspicion. Listed below are the major divisions we use to divide patients who present with chest pain.

ANATOMY

There are a number of clinically important structures in the chest. Clinically, we divide the chest into the superficial structures such as skin, subcutaneous tissue, muscle and ribs, and sternum. The deep compartment is everything deep to the parietal pleura, i.e., lungs, heart, esophagus, etc. (Fig. 2-1). This is very important because a large number of clinical cases of chest pain result from chest wall pathology which, for the most part, is less clinically significant than deeper chest pain that might be seen from an MI. In cases where the superficial structures are involved with disease states that present with chest pain, the pain will tend to be somatic, i.e., well localized. Thus, in a patient who presents with chest pain from a fractured rib, the pain will be sharp and well localized over the area of the fracture. On the other hand, the pain of an MI tends to be dull, crushing, and at times poorly localized. This is termed *visceral* pain and is carried by nerves that enter the spinal cord at multiple levels, resulting in a poorly localized pain. In the posterior mediastinum we encounter the esophagus and aorta. Aortic dissection, which we will learn about shortly, often results in bleeding into the retro-mediastinal space, which

Figure 2-1. Diagram of topographical anatomy of the chest in English and Spanish.

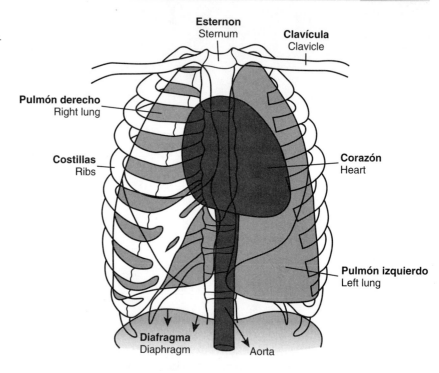

often presents clinically as severe back pain. Keep these anatomic relationships in mind when evaluating a patient with chest pain.

DIFFERENTIAL DIAGNOSIS OF CHEST PAIN

Cardiovascular ischemic
- MI
- Angina

Cardiovascular non-ischemic
- Aortic dissection
- Pericarditis

Non-cardiovascular
- Gastrointestinal
  - Esophageal (spasm, reflux, esophagitis)
  - Cholecystitis/choledocholithiasis
  - Peptic ulcer
  - Pancreatitis
- Pulmonary
  - Pulmonary embolism
  - Pneumothorax
  - Pneumonia
  - Pleuritis

- Musculoskeletal/connective tissue
    - Costochondritis
    - Sterno-clavicular arthritis
    - Herpes zoster (shingles)
    - Trauma (rib fracture, chest wall contusion)
- Panic disorder

APPROACH TO A PATIENT WITH CHEST PAIN

Remember—this line of questioning also is used for patients with abdominal pain, back pain, etc.

OBSERVATION

Just look to see how the patient is presenting. This is an often overlooked art in the hurried clinical practice of today but it is of incredible value in medicine. When one is seeing 20 people with chest pain during a 12-hour shift in a busy emergency room, this acquired skill will allow you to prioritize. For example, does the patient look like he or she is in acute distress or not? Is the patient clutching his or her chest? Is the patient gasping for air? Is the patient sweating or does he or she "look" sick? You can almost diagnose a patient by just observing. If the answer is "yes" to any of these questions, then you will need to work fast. The patient may have a life-threatening cardiac or pulmonary problem such as MI, aortic dissection, pneumothorax, or pulmonary embolus. These four etiologies of chest pain are the four life-threatening causes you have to rule in or out immediately, for if you miss any one of these, it could result in serious consequences. Rapid evaluation and monitoring will be crucial if any one of these four is suspected.

HISTORY

Ask a lot of open-ended questions so the patient can describe the pain. Once a basic description of the chest pain is given by the patient, it's now important to ask focused questions to narrow down the possible etiology.

As will be seen in subsequent chapters, *these are important questions when characterizing any pain.* Keep this in mind when reading the subsequent chapters.

- **The quality of pain**
    - On a scale of one to ten, ten being the worst pain of your life, how would you describe the pain you have right now? (Severe, excruciating pain, 9/10 or 10/10, may indicate aortic dissection.)
    - Describe the pain to me.
    - Does the pain feel like a squeezing/burning/tearing/sharp or dull pain? (Dull, pressure-like chest pain is more typical of an MI [visceral innervation], while sharp pain is more typical of chest wall pathology such as pleuritis or costochondritis [somatic innervation].)
    - Does the pain prevent you from doing things you normally do? (Angina is present with activity, thus this may limit the patient's activity.)

- **The location of the pain**
  - Point to the location of the pain.
  - Is the pain diffuse or localized? (The pain of visceral origin is poorly localized, while that of somatic origin is localized often by the patient pointing with one finger.)
  - Is the pain localized to the skin or breast bone?
  - Can the pain be reproduced by palpation or putting pressure on that location? (Pain to palpation is typical of chest wall disease versus a cardiac or pulmonary etiology.)
- **The radiation of the pain (where does the pain move)**
  - Is the pain in one location or does it radiate to other places?
  - Do you have any lower jaw, neck, or teeth pain? (Cardiac pain may radiate to the left arm or jaw or teeth.)
  - Do you have any tingling or numbness in your arms or hands?
  - Does the pain move to your back or shoulder blade? (Aortic dissection typically radiates to the back, while cholecystitis radiates to the scapula.)
  - Do you have any stomach pain? (Abdominal pathology such as gall bladder disease or pancreatitis may present predominately with chest pain.)
- **The duration of the chest pain**
  - Are you having chest pain now?
  - Is the pain constant or does it come and go? (Angina comes and goes related to activity, while an acute MI presents with constant pain.)
  - Did the pain just start today or has it been going on for some time? (Acute onset of pain is more likely to be life-threatening versus the chest pain that has been present for a longer period of time and that has not changed.)
  - When the pain does come, how long does it last? (The pain of angina is of short duration and corresponds to ceasing of a strenuous activity.)
- **Precipitating or relieving factors**
  - What makes the pain worse or what makes it better? (Pain of gallbladder origin is frequently exacerbated by fatty foods.)
  - Does exercise or exertion cause the pain? (Typical of cardiac pain.)
  - Does stress or anxiety bring on the pain?
  - Is the pain associated with meals? (Typical of abdominal pathology such as cholecystitis or pancreatitis.)
  - Does lying down or bending forward relieve the pain? (Bending forward often helps lessen the pain of pancreatitis.)
  - Is pain associated with deep breathing or coughing? (Typical of pneumonia and/or pleuritis, i.e., inflammation of the pleura.)
- **Associated symptoms**
  - Do you have shortness of breath with the pain? (Pneumonia, pneumothorax, or pulmonary embolus.)
  - Do you have sweating? (MI related to release of epinephrine.)
  - Do you have any lightheadedness or feel dizzy? (Sign of inadequate cardiac output or hypoxemia.)

- Do you have a cough? Are you coughing up anything? (Pneumonia—yellow sputum, pulmonary embolus—blood.)
- Do you have a fever? (Pneumonia)
- Did you hurt yourself or fall recently? (Chest wall trauma, rib fracture.)
- Do you recall any trauma to the chest area?
- Do you feel nervous or anxious? (MI, pulmonary embolus, pneumothorax, aortic dissection, panic disorder.)
- Do you have an overwhelming feeling of imminent doom or that something "bad" is about to happen? (Typical in patients with one of the four life-threatening causes of chest pain, but may be seen in panic disorder.)

Once you have asked the necessary questions, you will now be able to determine if this problem is acute or chronic. You will have a good feeling as to whether this pain reflects stable or unstable disease. Studies have shown that in 80% of patients, chest pain is of a noncardiovascular origin. To help predict the probability of possible cardiovascular disease, it is important to identify risk factors. You need to find out the patient's past medical history, social history, and family history. Risk factors for cardiac disease that will be important to know are:

- How old is the patient?
- Does he or she smoke?
- Any history of angina, hypertension, diabetes?
- What medications is he/she taking?
- Any history of heart attacks or cardiac catheterization procedures?
- Any history of open heart surgery?
- Is there a history of peripheral vascular disease? (If there is atherosclerosis in the peripheral arterial tree, there is also coronary artery disease.)
- Any history of high cholesterol?
- Does the patient use cocaine or other recreational drugs? (Cocaine increases oxygen demand of the heart, producing MI in relatively young patients and cardiac arrhythmias.)
- Any family history of heart disease?
- Have any family members died from heart disease? If so, how old were they when they passed away?
- Any recent colds or flu-like illnesses? (Viral cardiomyopathy may follow a seemingly mild viral disease.)

Remember that patients who present with chronic and recurring pain, without any real change in symptom pattern, are less likely to be emergent. For these patients, a differential diagnosis may include stable angina, gastrointestinal origin of the chest pain, or musculoskeletal pain. The patients to worry about are the ones who describe their pain as acute, i.e., recent onset, severe, progressive, unremitting. Further questioning may reveal a history of cardiovascular disease, a strong family history of atherosclerotic heart disease, or other risk factors for cardiac disease including smoking, hypertension, and diabetes.

Remember the detail of the history will depend on how urgent (i.e., how stable is your patient?) it is to arrive at the diagnosis.

FOCUSED PHYSICAL EXAM

1. **Check vital signs**. Any abnormality in blood pressure (BP), pulse (P), and respiratory rate (RR) may be a sign of a serious problem. Remember Airway, Breathing, and Circulation have to be addressed before the exam continues. For example, if the patient is tachypnic with shallow, labored breathing, you might have to intubate this patient to provide adequate oxygenation prior to proceeding.

2. **Check for jugular venous distension (JVD)**. Elevated jugular venous pressure should warn you of possible heart failure due to an MI (Fig. 2-2). Tension pneumothorax will also demonstrate this finding. This is due to inadequate blood return to the heart due to high pressures transmitted to the mediastinum from the pleural space, which is usually under negative pressure but due to the pneumothorax is converted to a high pressure zone (Fig. 2-3).

3. **Palpate for chest wall tenderness**. If deep palpation reproduces the pain, it is likely musculoskeletal versus cardiac or pulmonary.

4. **Assess heart sounds**. It's important to auscultate correctly, listening carefully for any abnormal sounds. An S3 or S4 heart sound may indicate ventricular wall non-compliance seen in congestive heart failure (CHF). Heart murmurs are indicative of abnormal valvular function. A rub is indicative of inflammation of the pericardial sac seen in pericarditis.

5. **Perform lung exam**. Listen carefully for any abnormalities. New onset of wheezing or rales (crackles) may indicate pulmonary edema secondary to an MI or heart condition. Friction rubs may indicate pleurisy, infection, or possible pulmonary embolism.

6. **Perform abdominal exam**. A thorough upper abdominal exam is important to check to see if the chest pain could be of gastrointestinal origin. Sometimes patients describe chest pain from cholecystitis, duodenal ulcer disease, and/or pancreatitis (all upper abdominal organs). An abdominal exam may reveal the true source of the pain. Of interest, at times an MI may present as upper abdominal pain, thus you can see the great cross-over in upper abdominal organ innervation and cardiac innervation.

7. **Extremity edema**. Check for pedal edema bilaterally (Fig. 2-4). This may be an indication of heart failure and underlying cardiac disease. Abnormal

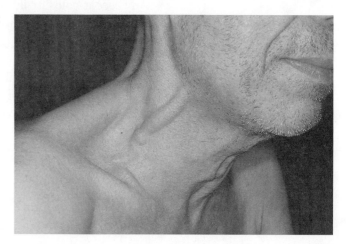

Figure 2-2. Jugular venous distension. (From Swartz M: *Textbook of Physical Diagnosis*, ed 5. Philadelphia, WB Saunders, 2005.)

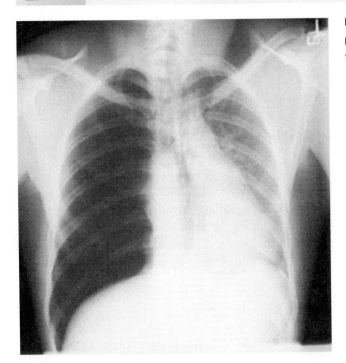

Figure 2-3. Note shift of the heart to the left due to right tension pneumothorax. Also note complete absence of vascular marking on the right side due to total collapse of the right lung.

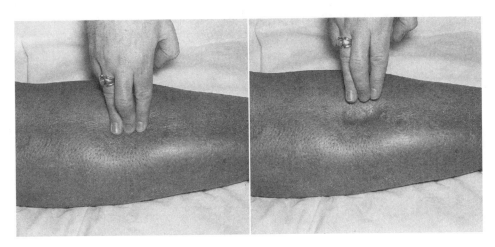

Figure 2-4. Pedal edema in a patient with CHF. (From Swartz M: *Textbook of Physical Diagnosis*, ed 5. Philadelphia, WB Saunders, 2005.)

swelling of one leg needs to be worked up for possible deep vein thrombosis, which may be the site from which a pulmonary embolus might arise, which would require an ultrasound of that leg to visualize the venous abnormalities. Bilateral edema often reflects CHF, producing a high hydrostatic pressure in the leg veins in relation to oncotic pressure resulting in fluid leaving the venous space to enter the interstitial space producing edema.

POSSIBLE INITIAL LABORATORY TESTS IN PATIENTS WITH CHEST PAIN

1. **Electrocardiogram (ECG or EKG):** If you even remotely suspect a cardiac origin for the pain, get an ECG. This test will demonstrate any evidence of ischemia as occurs with an acute MI as well as rhythm abnormalities that also may accompany an MI or be of primary etiology. Remember an abnormal cardiac rhythm, i.e., non-sinus rhythm, may result in a rapid

ventricular response increasing heart rate and oxygen demand of the myocardium. This may result in chest pain similar to that seen in an acute MI.

2. **Arterial blood gas**: If indicated, to check for hypoxemia indicative of pulmonary problems such as pulmonary embolus or pneumonia.

3. **Chest X-ray**: To rule out pneumothorax, pneumonia, heart failure, or skeletal fractures. Abnormalities in mediastinal shape and size may indicate heart or aortic abnormalities. Free mediastinal air may be visualized, indicating possible esophageal rupture.

4. **Blood tests**: Typical tests for chest pain when MI is even remotely suspected include: troponins, creatine kinase (biomarkers for heart disease), and arterial blood gas (ABG) to check for arterial oxygen and carbon dioxide partial pressures. In pulmonary embolus and pneumonia the oxygen levels are typically low. PH and bicarbonate levels are also obtained on ordering an ABG.

CASE 1: MYOCARDIAL INFARCTION

CHIEF COMPLAINT

Mr. Henderson is a 64-year-old male patient with acute onset of chest pain for four hours' duration.

HISTORY

	English	Spanish Formal	Spanish Informal
	Mr. Henderson, my name is Claudia López, I am a third year medical student working with Dr. Rap. I need to ask you some questions about what brought you here today.	Hola, Sr. Henderson, mi nombre es Claudia López. Soy estudiante de medicina de tercer año que trabaja con el Dr. Rap. Necesito hacerle unas preguntas sobre la razón por la que vino hoy.	Hola, señor Henderson, me llamo Claudia López. Soy estudiante de medicina de tercer año. Trabajo con el Dr. Rap y le voy a hacer unas preguntas sobre el motivo por el cual vino hoy.
Q.	How old are you?	¿Qué edad tiene?	¿Cuántos años tiene?
A.	I am sixty-four years old.	Tengo sesenta y cuatro años.	Sesenta y cuatro.
Q.	Are you currently having chest pain now?	¿Tiene dolor de pecho en este momento?	¿Le duele el pecho ahora?
A.	Yes.	Sí.	Sí.
Q.	How would you describe the pain?	¿Cómo describiría el dolor?	¿Cómo es el dolor?
A.	It feels like a squeezing pain around my chest.	Es un dolor opresivo, como que me apretaran alrededor del pecho.	Siento como que me apretaran el pecho.
Q.	When did the pain start?	¿Cuándo comenzó el dolor?	¿Cuándo empezó?
A.	About four hours ago, when I was mowing the lawn.	Hace como cuatro horas, cuando estaba cortando el césped.	Hace cuatro horas, cuando estaba cortando zacate (*monte*).

	English	Spanish Formal	Spanish Informal
Q.	Are you having any shortness of breath?	¿Tiene dificultad para respirar?	¿Siente que le falta el aire?
A.	Yes, I am. It's hard to breathe.	Sí, es difícil respirar.	Sí, me cuesta respirar.
Q.	Have you ever had pain like this before?	¿Alguna vez ha tenido un dolor semejante?	¿Alguna vez ha tenido un dolor parecido (*como este*)?
A.	I have had a similar pain but it went away when I stopped and rested. This time when I stopped working, the pain continued.	He tenido un dolor semejante, pero se me alivió cuando me detuve y descansé. Esta vez cuando dejé de trabajar, el dolor continuó.	Tuve un dolor parecido, pero se quitó cuando dejé de trabajar y descansé. Pero esta vez, cuando dejé de trabajar, el dolor no se quitó.
Q.	Where is the pain located? Can you describe it?	¿Dónde es el dolor? ¿Lo puede describir?	¿Dónde le duele? ¿Cómo es el dolor?
A.	Well, it's a tightness, a pressure around the center of my chest.	Bueno, es un apretazón, una presión en el centro del pecho.	Es como un apretazón en la mitad del pecho.
Q.	Does it move anywhere?	¿Se mueve para alguna parte?	¿Se le mueve?
A.	Yes, it moves down my left arm.	Sí, se mueve para abajo por el brazo izquierdo.	Sí, se me va para abajo por el brazo izquierdo.
Q.	Have you been sweating?	¿Ha estado sudando?	¿Ha sudado?
A.	Yes, I am sweating.	Sí, estoy sudando.	Sí.
Q.	Have you had any abdominal pain?	¿Ha tenido dolor en el abdomen?	¿Ha tenido dolor de panza?
A.	No, I have had no abdominal pain.	No, no he tenido dolor en el abdomen (*estómago*).	No.
Q.	Have you had nausea or vomiting with the chest pain?	¿Ha tenido náuseas o vómito con el dolor de pecho?	¿Ha tenido ganas de vomitar o vomitó con el dolor de pecho?
A.	I am really nauseous and sweaty. I have not thrown up but I feel like I am going to.	Tengo muchas náuseas y estoy sudando. No he vomitado, pero siento como que lo voy a hacer.	Tengo muchas ganas de vomitar y estoy sudando. No he vomitado, pero tengo muchas ganas.
Q.	Does anything make the pain worse or better?	¿Hay algo que hace mejor o peor el dolor?	¿Hay algo que mejora o empeora el dolor?
A.	I took a nitroglycerin tablet and it improved a little but then returned just as bad as before. If I am active, it gets worse.	Tomé una tableta de nitroglicerina y mejoró un poco, pero después regresó tan fuerte como antes. Si estoy activo, el dolor empeora.	Me tomé una nitroglicerina y mejoró, pero después me pegó recio otra vez. Si hago ejercicio, es peor.
Q.	Do you have any medical illnesses?	¿Tiene algún otro problema de salud o enfermedad?	¿Tiene otra enfermedad?
A.	Well, I have had a history of hypertension for about thirty years. I also have high cholesterol, but it's been under control with medication. I am also diabetic.	Bueno, he padecido de hipertensión desde hace treinta años. También tengo el colesterol alto, pero ha estado bajo control con la medicina. Además soy diabético.	Tengo la presión alta desde hace treinta años. También el colesterol alto, pero tomo la medicina para controlarlo. También tengo diabetes.
Q.	How long have you been diabetic?	¿Desde hace cuánto padece de la diabetes?	¿Desde cuándo tiene diabetes?
A.	Oh, about twenty years.	Pues, desde hace veinte años.	Como desde hace veinte años.
Q.	What medications are you taking?	¿Qué tratamiento tiene?	¿Qué medicina está tomando?
A.	I take lisinopril for my hypertension. I also take Lipitor for my cholesterol. For my diabetes, I am on metformin.	Tomo Lisinopril para la hipertensión. También tomo Lipitor para el colesterol. Para la diabetes, tomo Metformin.	Tomo Lisinopril para la presión alta, Lipitor para el colesterol y Metformin para la diabetes.

	English	Spanish Formal	Spanish Informal	Continued
Q.	Any family history of heart disease?	¿Alguien en su familia ha padecido de enfermedades del corazón?	¿Algún familiar ha padecido del corazón?	
A.	Yes, my brother passed away of a heart attack at sixty. My father died of a heart attack at fifty-five. That's about it.	Sí, mi hermano falleció de un ataque del corazón a los sesenta. Mi papá murió de un ataque del corazón a los cincuenta y cinco. Creo que eso es todo.	Sí, mi hermano y mi papá murieron de ataques al corazón. Mi hermano tenía sesenta años cuando murió, y papá, cincuenta y cinco.	
Q.	Do you smoke or drink?	¿Toma licor o fuma cigarrillos?	¿Fuma o toma?	
A.	I don't drink but I do smoke about half a pack a day. I have been smoking now for about twenty years.	No tomo licor pero me fumo como medio paquete al día. He fumado como por alrededor de veinte años.	No tomo, pero me fumo como medio paquete diario. He fumado como veinte años.	
Q.	Have you done any recreational drugs like cocaine or marijuana?	¿Alguna vez ha usado drogas como cocaína o marihuana?	¿Alguna vez ha usado cocaína o marihuana?	
A.	Oh no, never touched the stuff.	No, nunca he tocado esas cosas.	No.	

With this type of presentation, it is important to go directly to the critical questions. Here, MI should be high on the list of the differential diagnosis (things that the patient might have). You need to work quickly when a patient like this presents with acute onset of chest pain. Time is of the essence. Based on the patient's clinical presentation as well as history of risk factors and family history, a cardiac origin of the chest pain is likely. The physical exam and labs become crucial to assist in making a diagnosis and directing proper treatment.

PATHOPHYSIOLOGY

Myocardial ischemia occurs when oxygen demand to a particular part of the heart is not met. The problem usually arises because of insufficient coronary artery blood flow due to a blockage in the artery from atherosclerosis. The lack of oxygen to myocardial cells forces them to switch from aerobic to anaerobic metabolism, resulting in metabolic, mechanical, and electrical abnormalities. Angina pectoris is the most common manifestation of ischemia. Patients may present with chest pain that comes and goes for years before an MI occurs. Conversely, a patient may present with an MI without any prior history of angina. As a patient increases physical activity, the oxygen demand increases in the myocardial cells. If that demand is not met, ischemia and subsequent pain ensues. When the activity stops, oxygen demand by the heart is reduced, causing the pain to improve.

Occasionally, the pain may radiate or move to the left arm, jaw, neck, and/or back. This type of pain is termed referred pain. Pain from the heart is felt in various regions of the body. The reason for the 'referral' of visceral pain is the lack of a dedicated sensory pathway to the brain for information concerning the internal organs. The sensory neurons from the viscera enter the spinal cord and converge on other nerves as they move up toward the brain. This convergence can send mixed signals to the brain. Unfortunately, the brain cannot sort out the exact location of where the pain is coming from and so pain is felt in multiple areas (Fig. 2-5). Remember, in female patients often an atypical presentation is common; often the only complaint in this group of patients may be fatigue and vague nondescript chest or abdominal pain.

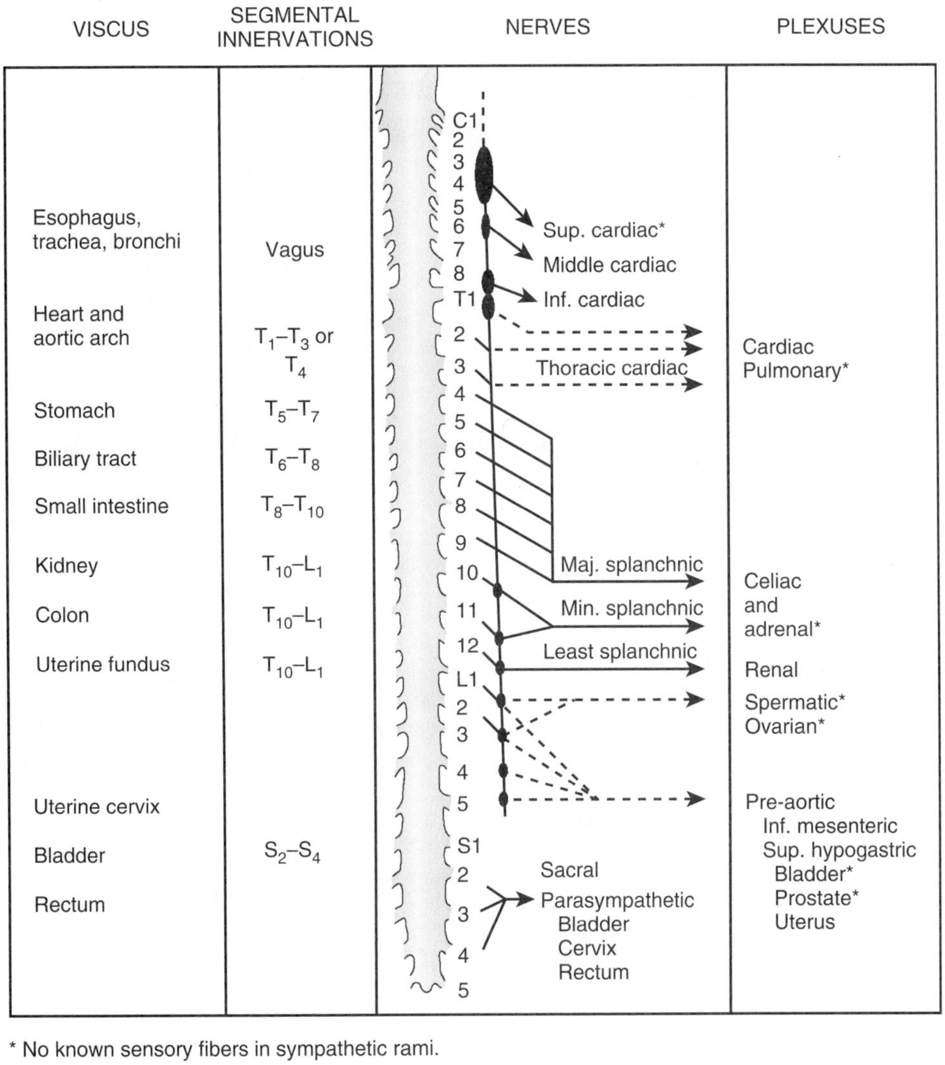

VISCUS	SEGMENTAL INNERVATIONS	NERVES	PLEXUSES

		C1	
		2	
		3	
		4	
Esophagus, trachea, bronchi	Vagus	5 — Sup. cardiac*	
		6	
		7 — Middle cardiac	
		8	
Heart and aortic arch	T_1–T_3 or T_4	T1 — Inf. cardiac	
		2	Cardiac Pulmonary*
		3 — Thoracic cardiac	
Stomach	T_5–T_7	4	
		5	
Biliary tract	T_6–T_8	6	
		7	
Small intestine	T_8–T_{10}	8	
		9	
Kidney	T_{10}–L_1	10 — Maj. splanchnic	Celiac and adrenal*
Colon	T_{10}–L_1	11 — Min. splanchnic	
		12 — Least splanchnic	
Uterine fundus	T_{10}–L_1	L1	Renal
		2	Spermatic* Ovarian*
		3	
		4	
Uterine cervix		5	Pre-aortic Inf. mesenteric Sup. hypogastric
Bladder	S_2–S_4	S1	Bladder* Prostate*
		2 — Sacral	Uterus
Rectum		3 — Parasympathetic Bladder Cervix Rectum	
		4	
		5	

* No known sensory fibers in sympathetic rami.

Figure 2-5. Visceral nerves enter the spinal cord at multiple levels versus somatic nerves. (From Townsend C: *Sabiston Textbook of Surgery*, ed 17. Philadelphia, WB Saunders, 2004.)

FOCUSED PHYSICAL EXAM

English	Spanish Formal	Spanish Informal
Mr. Henderson, can you remove your shirt and undershirt and put on this gown? I am concerned you may be having a heart attack so we will work fast. One of the nurses will be drawing blood and performing an ECG, a test of the heart, while I do the physical exam. We will also be giving you nasal oxygen and we will give you something for the pain right away.	Sr. Henderson, ¿se puede quitar la camisa y la camiseta y ponerse esta bata? Estoy preocupado porque es posible que usted tenga un ataque del corazón, así que vamos a trabajar rápidamente. Una de las enfermeras le va a sacar sangre y le va a hacer un examen del corazón que se llama electrocardiograma (ECG), mientras yo le hago un examen físico. También le vamos a dar oxígeno por la nariz y algo para el dolor en este momento.	Sr. Henderson, por favor quítese la camisa y la camiseta y se pone esta bata. Pienso que es posible que usted tenga un ataque del corazón, así que vamos a trabajar rápido. Una enfermera le va a sacar sangre y le va a hacer un electrocardiograma, mientras yo lo examino. Le vamos a poner oxígeno y darle algo para el dolor.

When we suspect a possible MI, a number of things occur simultaneously due to the urgency of the problem. Often, while we are doing the physical exam, someone is drawing blood for lab tests as well as applying chest leads for performing an ECG, applying nasal oxygen, and giving morphine to alleviate the pain. Aspirin is also given.

English	Spanish Formal	Spanish Informal
I am going to check your blood pressure and pulse again. Next, I am going to listen to your heart and lungs.	Le voy a tomar el pulso y la presión arterial otra vez. Después, le voy a escuchar el corazón y los pulmones.	Le voy tomar la presión y el pulso una vez más. Después, le voy a oír el corazón y los pulmones.
Now, I am going to examine your abdomen. I will be pressing softly. Just let me know if anything hurts or feels uncomfortable.	Ahora le voy a examinar el abdomen. Voy a presionarlo suavemente. Dígame si le duele o si siente alguna molestia.	Le voy a examinar la panza. Dígame si le duele o siente alguna molestia cuando lo toco.
Now the nurse is going to put on some sticky patches to monitor your heart. The nurse is also going to put something on your index finger. This is a monitor that will let us know if you're getting enough oxygen (this is termed a pulse oximeter).	Ahora la enfermera le va a poner unos parches en el pecho para monitorear su corazón. La enfermera también le va a colocar un aparato en el dedo índice. Es un monitor que nos va a indicar si usted está recibiendo suficiente oxígeno (se llama oxímetro de pulso).	Ahora la enfermera le va a poner unos parches en el pecho para conectarlo a una máquina que nos va a decir cómo esta su corazón. También le va a poner un aparato en el dedo para ver si está recibiendo suficiente oxígeno.
We are going to draw some blood to check if you have had a heart attack, and get a chest x-ray to check your lungs and heart.	Le vamos a sacar una muestra de sangre para ver si ha tenido un ataque del corazón, y una radiografía de tórax para evaluar los pulmones y el corazón.	Le vamos a sacar un poco de sangre para ver si ha tenido un ataque del corazón, y una radiografía de pecho para ver cómo están los pulmones y el corazón.

PHYSICAL EXAM RESULTS

- BP in left arm 148/98, P 116, RR 30, Temp. 36.7° C.
- **General appearance**: Patient is sitting up in bed having some mild shortness of breath. He appears in mild distress.
- **Lungs**: Rales are present at both bases. Good clear breath bilaterally in the middle and upper lung fields.
- **Cardiovascular**: Regular rate and rhythm, normal S1 and S2. Patient has a S4 gallop. No murmurs are heard. Mild jugular venous distention is present.
- **Abdomen**: Obese, soft, nontender, nondistended. Bowel sounds are present. Liver is normal size.
- **Extremities**: No clubbing, cyanosis, or pedal edema is present.

Based on the above findings, an MI with CHF is likely. It is always wise to put on top of the differential diagnosis the disease most likely to harm the patient if not diagnosed. The heart failure is diagnosed by the bilateral basilar rales, which occur due to cardiac or pump failure causing an elevated end diastolic volume in the left atrium. This increased left atrial pressure is transmitted to the pulmonary capillaries causing an increase in hydrostatic pressure and extravasation of fluid into the pulmonary alveoli causing rales. The jugular venous distention also points to heart failure (elevation in right atrial pressure), as does the S4 on cardiac exam indicating non-compliance of the left ventricle. The extra sound is the blood in the left atria hitting the wall of the noncompliant ventricle at the end of diastole. A pulmonary problem such as pneumonia is unlikely due to the symmetry of the rales or crackles and the fact that they occur at the bases. This finding is most likely due to CHF, as the bases of the lungs have the highest hydrostatic pressure since they are more dependent than the upper lobes. In pneumonia, the rales are typically localized over the area of pneumonia. Tension pneumothorax is ruled out by the presence of good breath sounds bilaterally. In a pneumothorax there is air in the pleural space occurring from a rupture of a part of the bronchial tree from trauma or spontaneously producing a decrease in breath sounds from collapse of the ipsilateral lung.

LAB RESULTS

- **CBC**: normal hemoglobin, hematocrit, WBC, and platelets.
- **Electrolytes**: WNL.
- **Troponins x 3**: elevated.
- **CK-MB**: levels elevated 4 hours after chest pain started.
- **ECG**: sinus tachycardia, elevated ST segment in inferior leads (Fig. 2-6).
- **Chest X-ray**: cardiomegaly (Fig. 2-7).

DIAGNOSIS

Myocardial infarction with congestive heart failure.

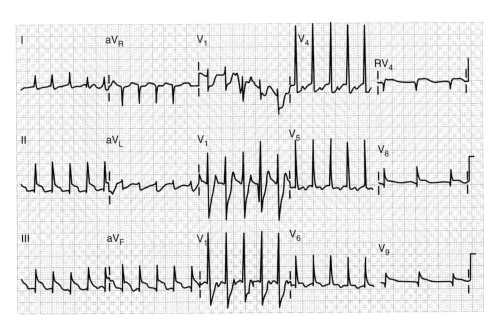

Figure 2-6. ECG showing an inferior MI. (From Marx J, Hockberger R, Walls R: *Rosen's Emergency Medicine: Concepts and Clinical Practice*, ed 6. Philadelphia, Mosby, 2006.)

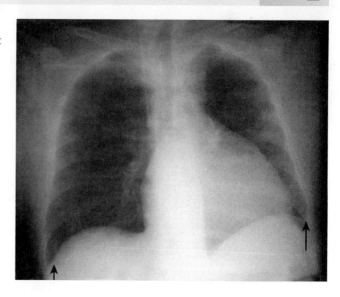

Figure 2-7. Chest x-ray showing CHF. Note cardiac enlargement, which should be less than half of the distance from one costophrenic angle to the other (*arrows*).

INITIAL MANAGEMENT

Based on the information gathered, it seems that our patient is experiencing a myocardial infarction. It now becomes important to monitor the patient to make sure no arrhythmia occurs. Arrhythmia is the major cause of death in early post-MI. The most common arrhythmia is ventricular fibrillation. A beta blocker is given usually to decrease cardiac contractility and rate, thus reducing oxygen consumption of the heart unless, as in this case, it is contraindicated due to heart failure. The standard management for this patient would be high flow oxygen, aspirin, and pain relief (usually morphine). Nitroglycerin sublingually is usually given in the ER Department. This vasodilator preferentially dilates the coronary arteries providing increased circulation to the ischemic heart.

(1) Oxygen

(2) Pain relief

(3) Nitroglycerin

(4) Emergent angiogram is indicated if continued ischemia occurs. Clinically this is assessed by the chest pain the patient is experiencing and the ECG. An angiogram is performed in such cases so that the narrowed coronary artery can be diagnosed and treated by dilating the artery with a balloon catheter placed usually through the femoral artery and putting in a stent to maintain patency of the coronary artery. This allows an increase in flow to the ischemic region of the heart without having to undergo open heart surgery in many cases.

(5) Thrombolytics: These are medications given to dissolve the thrombi or clot in the coronary arteries. They can be given systemically or directly into the coronary arteries during angiogram.

DISCUSSION OF MANAGEMENT WITH THE PATIENT

English	Spanish Formal	Spanish Informal
Mr. Henderson, all the tests that we have done point to the diagnosis of heart attack or myocardial infarction. That's the reason	Sr. Henderson, todas las pruebas que hemos hecho nos señalan el diagnóstico de ataque del corazón o infarto del miocardio. Esa es la	Sr. Henderson, las pruebas que le hemos hecho nos dicen que usted tuvo un ataque del corazón. Por eso fue que tuvo

English	Spanish Formal	Spanish Informal
for the chest pain you experienced this evening. Right now everything looks stable. We are giving you medication to improve the oxygen going to the heart. We are going to call the cardiologists to see you and they probably will want to get an arteriogram to see if there is a blockage in the arteries to the heart. If there is, they can sometimes put in medicines to unblock the arteries or a stent to open the artery up.	causa del dolor de pecho que usted experimentó esta noche. Por el momento, todo parece estable. Le estamos dando medicamentos para aumentar la cantidad de oxígeno que llega al corazón. Vamos a llamar a los cardiólogos para que lo examinen. Ellos probablemente van a querer hacerle una arteriografía para ver si existe un bloqueo de las arterias coronarias. Si existe bloqueo, ellos a veces le ponen unos medicamentos para remover la obstrucción o un *stent* (*pequeño tubo flexible*) para abrir la arteria.	dolor de pecho. Por el momento, todo parece bien. Le estamos dando medicinas para que le llegue más oxígeno al corazón. Vamos a llamar a los cardiólogos para que lo vean. Es posible que ellos quieran hacerle una arteriografía para ver si hay una obstrucción de las arterias del corazón. Si hay obstrucción, ellos pueden ponerle unas medicinas para quitar la obstrucción o un tubo pequeño, que se llama *stent*, para abrir la arteria.
Q. (Mr. Henderson): What is an angiogram?	(Sr. Henderson): ¿Qué es una arteriografía?	(Sr. Henderson): ¿Qué es una arteriografía?
A. (Dr. Rap): It's a procedure to look at the blood vessels of the heart. A heart attack is usually caused from closure or narrowing of the blood vessels in the heart. This procedure allows us to visualize these arteries and, if opening the arteries is needed to get more blood to the heart, they can do this at the time they do the angiogram.	(Dr. Rap): Es un procedimiento para ver los vasos sanguíneos del corazón. Un ataque del corazón generalmente es el resultado de una obstrucción o estrechamiento de los vasos sanguíneos en el corazón. Este procedimiento nos permite visualizar estas arterias y, si es necesario abrir las arterias para que llegue más sangre al corazón, ellos pueden hacerlo al mismo tiempo que hacen la angiografía.	(Dr. Rap): Bueno, es un examen para ver las arterias del corazón. Un ataque del corazón generalmente se debe a un taponamiento o estrechamiento de las arterias del corazón. La arteriografía nos ayuda a ver la parte de adentro de las arterias y, de ser necesario, a abrirlas un poco para que llegue más sangre al corazón.
Q. Do you have any other questions?	¿Tiene otras preguntas?	¿Tiene preguntas?
A. No, not right now.	No por el momento.	No por ahora.

CASE 2: COSTOCHONDRITIS

CHIEF COMPLAINT

Mrs. Silvia Gutierrez is a 68-year-old female with a past medical history of recent open heart surgery (quadruple bypass 6 months ago), who now comes to the ER with severe chest pain.

FOCUSED HISTORY

Again, this is a case where the patient could be experiencing a serious problem. A quick history and physical are needed to rule out a cardiac origin of the pain.

English	Spanish Formal	Spanish Informal
Hi, Mrs. Gutierrez, my name is Jesse McClellan. I am a third year medical student working with Dr. Jackson. I need to	Buenas tardes, Sra. Gutiérrez, me llamo Jesse McClellan. Soy un estudiante de medicina de tercer año. Trabajo con el Dr.	Hola, Sra. Gutiérrez, soy Jesse McClellan, estudiante de medicina de tercer año. Trabajo con el Dr. Jackson. Necesito

	English	Spanish Formal	Spanish Informal Continued
	ask you some questions about your problem.	Jackson. Necesito hacerle unas preguntas sobre su problema de salud.	hacerle unas preguntas sobre su problema.
Q.	What brings you to the emergency room today?	¿Por qué vino a la sala de emergencias hoy?	¿Por qué vino a emergencias?
A.	I am having chest pain.	Tengo dolor de pecho.	Estoy con dolor de pecho.
Q.	How old are you?	¿Qué edad tiene?	¿Cuántos años tiene?
A.	I am sixty-eight years old.	Tengo sesenta y ocho años.	Sesenta y ocho.
Q.	Are you currently having chest pain?	¿Tiene dolor de pecho en este momento?	¿Tiene dolor de pecho ahora?
A.	Yes, the pain is really bad.	Sí, me duele mucho.	Sí, bastante.
Q.	What does the pain feel like? Can you describe it?	¿Cómo siente el dolor? ¿Me lo puede describir?	¿Cómo es el dolor? ¿Lo puede describir?
A.	It's a sharp, stabbing pain.	Es un dolor agudo, punzante.	Es como una puñalada.
Q.	Where is the pain located? Can you point to it?	¿Dónde siente el dolor? ¿Me puede mostrar (señalar dónde le duele)?	¿Dónde le duele? ¿Me puede enseñar?
A.	Its right here in the center of my chest (pointing just lateral to the lateral border of the right upper sternum).	Es aquí, en el centro del pecho (señalando la zona lateral al borde lateral del esternón superior derecho).	Aquí, en el centro del pecho.
Q.	Does the pain move anywhere or does it stay in one spot?	¿El dolor se mueve a alguna otra parte o se queda en el mismo lugar?	¿Se le mueve para alguna otra parte o se queda en el mismo lugar?
A.	No, it stays in one spot.	No, se queda en el mismo lugar.	No, se queda en un lugar.
Q.	How long have you had this pain?	¿Cuánto tiempo ha tenido ese dolor?	¿Por cuánto tiempo lo ha tenido?
A.	It started two days ago as a vague pain and has been getting worse.	Comenzó hace dos días como una molestia y se ha hecho peor.	Desde hace dos días. Al principio sólo era una molestia y después empeoró.
Q.	What were you doing when the pain started?	¿Qué estaba haciendo cuando le comenzó el dolor?	¿Qué estaba haciendo cuando le empezó el dolor?
A.	Nothing really, I have been in bed for the past week with a real bad cold and have not really done anything.	Realmente nada. Había estado en cama toda la semana con un resfriado muy fuerte y no había hecho nada realmente.	Nada. Tenía una semana de estar en cama sin hacer nada con un resfrío muy fuerte.
Q.	What makes the pain worse and what makes it better?	¿Qué hace empeorar el dolor y qué lo hace mejorar?	¿Qué mejora o empeora el dolor?
A.	Well, I have been coughing for the past two weeks and coughing makes the pain worse. Taking a deep breath in makes it worse as well. Laying down makes the pain feel better.	Pues, he estado tosiendo las últimas dos semanas y la tos empeora el dolor. También cuando inspiro con fuerza me duele más. Cuando estoy acostado me siento mejor (se me alivia el dolor).	La tos empeora el dolor. También me duele más cuando respiro recio para adentro. Se me quita un poco cuando estoy acostada.
Q.	Are you short of breath?	¿Tiene dificultad para respirar?	¿Siente que le falta el aire?
A.	Yes, but it's because my nose is clogged up and I am still coughing up a lot of mucus.	Sí, pero es porque tengo la nariz tapada (bloqueada) y todavía estoy tosiendo un montón de flemas.	Sí, pero es porque estoy mormada (con congestión nasal) y todavía estoy tosiendo un montón de flemas (gargajos).
Q.	Do you have nausea or vomiting?	¿Tiene náusea o ha vomitado?	¿Tiene ganas de vomitar o ha vomitado?
A.	No.	No.	No.

English	Spanish Formal	Spanish Informal
Q. Have you had any heart problems in the past?	¿Alguna vez en el pasado ha tenido problemas del corazón?	¿Alguna vez ha tenido problemas con el corazón?
A. I had a heart attack about one year ago.	Tuve un ataque del corazón hace un año.	Tuve un ataque del corazón el año pasado.
Q. Did they admit you to the hospital?	¿La internaron en el hospital?	¿La ingresaron en el hospital?
A. Yes, I was admitted to the intensive care unit.	Sí, me internaron en la unidad de cuidados intensivos.	Sí, me internaron en cuidados intensivos.
Q. Did they do any procedures such as surgery to prevent another heart attack?	¿Le hicieron algún otro procedimiento, como cirugía, para prevenir otro ataque del corazón?	¿Le hicieron algún procedimiento, como una operación, para evitar otro ataque?
A. Yes, they did bypass surgery.	Sí, me hicieron una cirugía de derivación cardíaca.	Sí, me hicieron una operación de "bypass."
Q. Does this pain feel similar to the pain you felt when you had your heart attack?	¿El dolor de ahora es semejante al que sintió cuando tuvo el ataque cardíaco?	¿Este dolor se parece al que sintió cuando tuvo el ataque al corazón?
A. No. This is a sharp pain.	No. Este es un dolor agudo.	No, este dolor es como una punzada.
Q. Have you had chest pain since your last heart attack?	¿Ha tenido dolor de pecho desde el último ataque del corazón?	¿Ha tenido dolor en el pecho desde el último infarto?
A. No, I have had no chest pain until these last two days.	No, no he tenido dolor de pecho hasta estos últimos dos días.	No, no he tenido dolor hasta estos últimos dos días.
Q. Did you take anything for the pain?	¿Tomó alguna medicina para el dolor?	¿Tomó algo para el dolor?
A. Yes, when the pain first came on I took a nitroglycerin pill that I keep at home, but the pain did not go away immediately like when I have angina pain. The pain lasted for about an hour, then it went away after I took two ibuprofen. But of course at that time I decided to lie down. The pain returned the next morning and I again tried a nitro pill. The pain didn't go away, so I decided to come to the emergency room.	Sí, cuando sentí dolor por primera vez me tomé una píldora de nitroglicerina que tenía en casa, pero el dolor no se quitó inmediatamente como cuando tengo angina de pecho. El dolor me duró como una hora y se me quitó después de que tomé dos Ibuprofen. Pero por supuesto en ese momento decidí acostarme. El dolor regresó a la mañana siguiente y otra vez me tomé la píldora de nitroglicerina. Como el dolor no se me quitó, decidí venir al servicio de emergencias.	Sí, cuando sentí el dolor primero me tomé una nitroglicerina pero no se me quitó de una vez (*luego, luego*), como cuando tengo el dolor de pecho. Tuve dolor como una hora y se me quitó después de tomarme dos Ibuprofen y acostarme. Al día siguiente me desperté con el dolor y otra vez me tomé la nitroglicerina, pero no me hizo nada. Así que decidí venirme para emergencias.
Q. What medications are you taking?	¿Qué medicinas está tomando?	¿Qué está tomando?
A. I am only taking 20 mg of Propanolol, 25 mg of Lisinopril, and a baby aspirin.	Sólo estoy tomando veinte miligramos de Propanolol, veinticinco miligramos de Lisinopril, y una aspirina.	Veinte miligramos de Propanolol, veinticinco miligramos de Lisinopril, y una aspirina.
Q. Now, how long have you had this cold and what symptoms have you been experiencing?	Bien, ¿por cuánto tiempo ha tenido este resfriado y qué síntomas ha tenido?	¿Por cuánto tiempo ha estado resfriada y qué síntomas ha tenido?
A. Well, the cold actually started three weeks ago with a runny nose and then the cough started about two weeks ago. Now the mucus that is coming from my nose and lungs has become dark green/brown.	Pues el resfriado me comenzó hace tres semanas con mocos por la nariz. Después, hace dos semanas, me comenzó la tos. Ahora las flemas que me vienen de la nariz y los pulmones son verde-café oscuro.	El resfrío empieza hace tres semanas con mocos por la nariz. He tenido tos por dos semanas y ahora tengo flemas de color verde-café oscuro.
Q. Have you had any fever or chills?	¿Ha tenido fiebre o escalofríos?	¿Ha tenido calentura o escalofríos?
A. Yes, but today it has been normal.	Sí, pero hoy he estado normal.	Sí, pero hoy he estado bien.

	English	Spanish Formal	Spanish Informal	Continued
Q.	Have you taken anything for the cold?	¿Ha tomado alguna medicina para el resfriado?	¿Ha tomado algo para el resfriado?	
A.	Sudafed, but it hasn't touched it.	Sudafed, pero no me ha hecho nada.	Sudafed, pero no sirve.	
Q.	Do you smoke or have you ever smoked?	¿Fuma o alguna vez ha fumado cigarrillos?	¿Fuma o ha fumado?	
A.	I stopped smoking about a year ago. Prior to that, I smoked about two packs a day for about forty years.	Dejé de fumar hace un año. Antes de dejarlo, fumaba como dos paquetes al día. Fumé como cuarenta años.	Dejé de fumar hace un año. Antes me fumaba dos paquetes diarios. Fumé cuarenta años.	
Q.	Do you have any allergies to medication?	¿Es alérgico a alguna medicina?	¿Padece de alergias a alguna medicina?	
A.	Yes, penicillin.	Sí, a la penicilina.	Sí, a penicilina.	

FOCUSED PHYSICAL EXAM

Typically, in the emergent-urgent situation we omit a fair amount of the history initially to arrive quickly at a diagnosis. This information can be filled in later, after the acute situation is dealt with.

	English	Spanish Formal	Spanish Informal
	Ok, Mrs. Gutierrez, I need to perform a physical exam so I am going to ask you to remove everything from the waist up and put on this gown. I will step out while you undress and in the meantime the nurse is going to place the ECG leads on you to monitor your heart and the pulse oximeter on your finger to check your oxygen level. Once all this is done, I will return to finish the exam.	Bueno, Sra. Gutiérrez, necesito hacerle un examen físico, así que le voy a pedir que se quite toda la ropa de la cintura para arriba y que se ponga esta bata. Voy a salir mientras se desviste y a la vez la enfermera le va a colocar las guías del ECG para monitorear su corazón y el oxímetro en el dedo para ver cómo anda el nivel de oxígeno en su sangre. Una vez que hayamos hecho todo esto, voy a regresar para terminar el examen.	Sra. Gutiérrez, vamos a hacerle un examen físico. Por favor, quítese la ropa de la cintura para arriba y póngase esta bata. Voy a salir mientras se desviste. A la vez, la enfermera le va a poner las guías del ECG para ver cómo anda su corazón y el oxímetro para medir el nivel de oxígeno en la sangre. Una vez que le hayamos hecho esto, regresaré otra vez para terminar el examen.
	Now I am just going to listen to your heart and lungs. Then I will do a quick check of your eyes, ears, nose, and throat. (Due to the urgency of the situation, the lungs and heart are examined first in this case.)	Ahora le voy a escuchar el corazón y los pulmones. Después le voy a examinar los ojos, los oídos, la nariz y la garganta rápidamente. (Debido a la urgencia de la situación, los pulmones y el corazón son examinados primero en este caso)	Ahora voy a escuchar el corazón y los pulmones. Después le voy a examinar los ojos, los oídos, la nariz y la garganta.
Q.	Now you said initially that the pain was in the center of your chest. Can you point to the exact location?	Ahora, usted dijo inicialmente que el dolor era en el centro del pecho. ¿Puede enseñarme el lugar exacto donde le duele?	Al principio, usted dijo que el dolor era en el centro del pecho. ¿Puede enseñarme dónde le duele?
A.	It's right along my sternum. Right here.	Es junto al esternón. Aquí.	Es a la par del esternón. Aquí.
Q.	Tell me if you feel pain as I press down on your sternum.	Dígame si le duele cuando pongo presión en el esternón.	Dígame si le duele cuando le aprieto el esternón.
A.	Yes! That's painful when you do that.	Sí, me duele cuando hace eso.	Sí
Q.	Is it the same pain you have been experiencing?	¿Es el mismo dolor que ha estado sintiendo?	¿Es el mismo dolor que ha tenido?
A.	Yes!	¡Sí!	¡Sí!

	English	Spanish Formal	Spanish Informal
Q.	Now I am going to press down on your belly. You tell me if you feel the same pain.	Ahora le voy a poner presión sobre el abdomen. Dígame si siente lo mismo.	Ahora le voy a apretar la barriga. Dígame si siente igual.
A.	No, there is no pain.	No, no siento dolor.	No, no me duele.
Q.	Well, I want to run a few tests. We have already done the ECG. We are going to draw some blood and check to see if you are having any heart problems. Then I would like to get a chest x-ray to see if we can see anything abnormal. I am more concerned about a possible heart attack again, so we need to make sure these tests are completed. After they are done, I will return with the results.	Bien, quiero hacerle unos exámenes. Ya le hicimos un ECG. Le vamos a sacar sangre para ver si tiene algún problema del corazón. Después me gustaría tener una radiografía de tórax para ver si hay algo anormal. Lo que más me preocupa es la posibilidad de que haya tenido otro ataque del corazón. Por eso tenemos que estar seguros de completar estos exámenes. Después de hacerlos regresaré con los resultados.	Bueno, le vamos a hacer unos exámenes. Ya le hicimos el ECG. Le vamos a sacar sangre para ver si tiene algún problema de corazón. Después, una radiografía de pecho para ver si hay algo anormal. Lo que más me preocupa es la posibilidad de que haya tenido otro ataque del corazón. Así que tenemos que hacerle estos exámenes para estar seguros. Cuando tenga los resultados, regresaré.
A.	Ok, do whatever you need to do.	Está bien, haga lo que tenga que hacer.	Está bien.

PHYSICAL EXAM RESULTS

- **Vitals**: T 38.0° C, P 80, R 14, BP 148/86. Pulse Ox 98% on room air.
- **General**: Appears in no acute distress.
- **Lungs**: Occasional wheezes heard as well as bilateral rhonchi. No rales (crackles). Good breath sounds bilaterally.
- **CV**: Regular rate and rhythm. Normal S1 and S2. No S3 or S4 appreciated. No murmurs, gallops, clicks or rub noted. No JVD.
- **Abdomen**: Obese, soft, nontender, nondistended, no hepatosplenomegaly, and bowel sounds present.
- **Musculoskeletal**: Large scar present down sternum (location of recent open heart surgery). Incision site is clean, dry, and without erythema. Joint tenderness at the costochondral articulations of the left anterior chest wall near ribs 3, 4, and 5. Pain reproducible by deep palpation.

DIFFERENTIAL DIAGNOSIS

English	Spanish Formal	Spanish Informal
- Myocardial infarction - Musculoskeletal: costochondritis or rib fracture - Pneumonia - Pulmonary embolus	- Infarto del miocardio - Músculo-esquelético: costocondritis o fractura costal - Neumonía - Embolia pulmonar	- Ataque del corazón - Inflamación de la articulación del pecho o quebradura de costilla - Pulmonía - Embolia de pulmón

As we said before and will stress throughout this book, it is crucial to rule out life-threatening diseases first, even though they are less likely than some of the other possibilities. The pain our patient is experiencing does not appear to be of cardiac origin. It is different from her prior MI pain—it is localized, direct pressure reproduces the pain, and it was relieved by an anti-inflammatory and not by nitroglycerin. Although this still does not rule out a cardiac etiology, it makes it less likely. Women in particular often have very atypical symptoms when they present with a myocardial infarction. Often they present with fatigue, atypical chest pain or upper abdominal pain, and very vague symptoms. This patient has many risk factors for cardiac disease including age, smoking history, prior cardiac surgery, etc. Thus, an ECG is crucial, as are troponins. Pneumonia is a possibility with her productive cough and low grade fever. Her lung findings of occasional wheezes and rhonchi may be her baseline "normal" exam. Her many years of smoking may have produced chronic damage termed chronic obstructive pulmonary disease (COPD). A chest radiograph will be helpful in clarifying this. Due to her recent surgery, she is at risk for forming a deep venous clot and having the clot break off producing a pulmonary embolus. However, the hallmark of a pulmonary embolus is shortness of breath and hypoxia. Her respiratory rate is normal and her pulse oximeter, which measures oxygen saturation, is normal, essentially ruling out this disease. Most likely the pain is musculoskeletal, i.e., costochondritis, an inflammation of the costochondral junction or a rib fracture that may occur in the elderly, especially from vigorous coughing. This is more common in patients with osteoporosis, and is therefore seen in women more often than in men. The localized sharp pain that is reproducible by palpation on physical exam speaks to one of these etiologies.

LAB RESULTS

- **CBC**: normal hemoglobin, hematocrit, WBC, and platelets.
- **Electrolytes**: WNL.
- **Troponins x 3**: normal.
- **CK-MB**: normal.
- **ECG**: Normal. No change from previous ECG taken during patient's last hospitalization 6 months ago.
- **Chest X-ray**: Cardiomegaly, no change from 6 months ago. Hyperinflation of both lungs with flattening of the diaphragms consistent with COPD (Fig. 2-8). The chest x-ray reveals mild cardiomegaly. There is no infiltration indicative of pneumonia.

What do the Lab Tests Tell You?

Based on the lab data, it can be concluded that the chest pain is not cardiac in origin. Negative elevation of troponins and no change in the ECG rule out MI. The radiograph shows no obvious pneumonia and there is evidence of mild CHF. Given the patient's history of recent upper respiratory infection and chest pain reproducible by palpation, it can be concluded that this patient has costochondritis.

PATHOPHYSIOLOGY

Costochondritis is an inflammatory process of the costochondral or costosternal joints that causes localized pain and tenderness. Pain is reproducible by palpation. Any one of the seven costochondral junctions may be affected. Ninety percent of cases show multiple joints affected. The second to fifth costochondral junctions most commonly are involved.

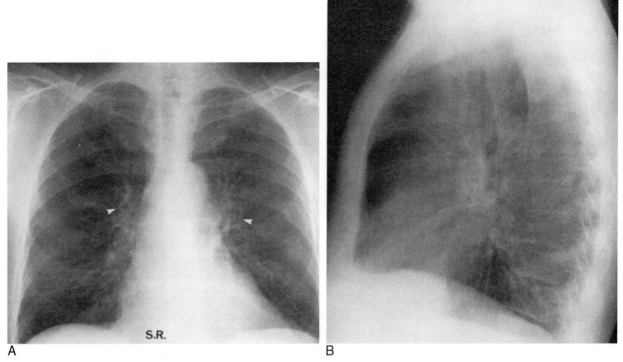

Figure 2-8. Chest x-ray showing COPD with no acute distress. Note the thickened bronchial walls viewed end-on in the right and left upper lobes (*arrows*). (From Fraser R, Muller N, Colman N, Pare P: *Fraser and Pare's Diagnosis of Diseases of the Chest*, ed 4. Philadelphia, WB Saunders, 1999.)

ASSESSMENT AND PLAN

Costochondritis. Treatment consists of non-steroidal anti-inflammatory agents such as ibuprofen. Sometimes the diagnosis may not be as black-and-white as this case. If your suspicion for a cardiac event is still present but labs show no indication of acute cardiac problems, it may be wise to admit the patient overnight to the hospital for cardiac monitoring. If no abnormalities are present after 24 hours, then the patient can be discharged home. In our case, the patient may be discharged home but with instructions to return to the ER if symptoms change for the worse.

DISCUSSION OF MANAGEMENT WITH THE PATIENT

English	Spanish Formal	Spanish Informal
Hi, Mrs. Gutierrez, I have some good news. The lab tests and ECG show that everything is fine in terms of your heart. Your troponin levels were normal, which indicates no active cardiac problems. The ECG results were the same as when you left the hospital six months ago. The chest pain that you feel is caused by an inflammation of the joints in the sternum. Your cough and upper respiratory symptoms are most	Sra. Gutiérrez, le tengo buenas noticias. Las pruebas de laboratorio y el ECG muestran que todo está bien con su corazón. El nivel de las troponinas fue normal, lo que indica que no tiene problemas activos en su corazón. Los resultados del ECG fueron semejantes a los que tenía cuando salió del hospital hace seis meses. El dolor de pecho que siente es causado por una inflamación de las articulaciones del esternón. La tos y los	Sra. Gutiérrez, tengo buenas noticias. Las pruebas de laboratorio y el ECG muestran que su corazón está bien. Los resultados del ECG son parecidos a los que tenía cuando salió del hospital hace seis meses. El dolor de pecho se debe a una inflamación de las articulaciones del esternón. La tos y el resfriado son por un virus. Si siente que está mejorando, es mejor no darle antibióticos por ahora.

English	Spanish Formal	Spanish Informal	Continued
likely caused by a virus and if you feel you are improving, we will hold off giving you antibiotics. I will write you a prescription for an antitussive medication which will help quiet your cough. This will also help to alleviate the chest pain.	síntomas respiratorios superiores posiblemente son de origen viral. Si siente que está mejorando, es mejor esperar y no darle antibióticos. Le voy a escribir una receta para una medicina antitusiva, le ayudará a calmar la tos. También le aliviará el dolor de pecho.	Le voy a dar una medicina para la tos. También le ayudará con el dolor de pecho.	
The anti-inflammatory agent that I want you to take for the joint chest pain is ibuprofen. I will write you a prescription for 800 mg tablets three times per day as needed for pain. You may also want to try to put a heating pad over the area, which may help. Avoid strenuous activity, especially any activity that causes you to twist your body. Please follow up with your primary care physician in one week to see how everything is going. If you are not feeling better in twenty-four hours, we need you to come back in to be seen or sooner if you start to feel worse. Do you have any questions?	El anti-inflamatorio que quiero que tome para el dolor de la articulación del pecho es ibuprofén. Le voy a escribir una receta para que tome ochocientos miligramos tres veces al día mientras esté con dolor. También puede ponerse compresas calientes (toallas calientes) sobre el área afectada, le pueden ayudar. Evite actividades pesadas (arduas), especialmente cualquier actividad en la que tenga que doblar el cuerpo. Por favor, consulte con su médico de cabecera dentro de una semana para ver cómo sigue. Si no se siente bien en veinticuatro horas o si comienza a sentirse peor, necesitamos que regrese para verla. ¿Tiene alguna pregunta?	Quiero que tome Ibuprofen para la inflamación de la articulación del pecho. Le voy a recetar ochocientos miligramos tres veces al día. También puede ponerse toallas (paños) de agua caliente sobre el pecho donde le duele, le va a ayudar. Evite hacer trabajo pesado, especialmente actividades en las que tenga que doblar el cuerpo. Visite a su médico dentro de una semana para ver cómo sigue. Si no se siente bien para mañana o si se pone peor, tiene que volver para ver la otra vez. ¿Tiene preguntas?	
A. No, I am actually kind of relieved to know it's not a heart problem. OK, well, I think you have answered all my questions and concerns. Thank you.	No, en realidad me siento mejor de saber que el problema no es del corazón. Está bien, yo creo que usted me ha contestado todas mis preguntas y preocupaciones. ¡Muchas gracias!	No, me siento muy bien de saber que no es un problema del corazón. No tengo preguntas, usted ya me dijo todo lo que necesitaba saber. ¡Le agradezco mucho!	
OK, Mrs. Gutierrez, I hope this works for you, take care.	Está bien, Sra. Gutiérrez, espero que todo salga bien. Cuídese mucho.	Muy bien, Sra. Gutiérrez, espero que todo salga bien. Cuídese mucho.	

One of the keys to dealing with patients with chest pain is clear instructions about follow-up if they are discharged from clinic or the ER. It is crucial they be seen back again either in the ER or by their primary care giver if symptoms get worse. Obviously, if they improve, they can follow up with their primary doctor.

CASE 3: ESOPHAGEAL SPASM

CHIEF COMPLAINT

Mrs. Gloria Duarte is a 39-year-old female who presents with a three-day history of chest pain to the Medical Clinic.

HISTORY

English	Spanish Formal	Spanish Informal
Hi, Mrs. Duarte, my name is Bob Parra, I am a third-year medical student working with Dr. Ortiz. I need to ask you some questions about your problem.	Hola, Sra. Duarte, mi nombre es Bob Parra. Soy un estudiante de medicina de tercer año. Trabajo con el Dr. Ortíz. Necesito hacerle unas preguntas sobre su problema.	Sra. Duarte, me llamo Bob Parra. Soy un estudiante de medicina de tercer año y trabajo con el Dr. Ortíz. Necesito hacerle unas preguntas.

English	Spanish Formal	Spanish Informal
Q. How old are you?	¿Qué edad tiene?	¿Cuántos años tiene?
A. I am 39 years old.	Tengo treinta y nueve años.	Treinta y nueve.
Q. Are you currently having chest pain?	¿Tiene dolor de pecho en este momento?	¿Tiene dolor de pecho?
A. Yes.	Sí.	Sí.
Q. How long have you had this pain?	¿Desde hace cuánto tiempo tiene dolor?	¿Desde cuándo tiene dolor?
A. Off and on for three days now.	Desde hace tres días el dolor me viene y se me va.	Viene y se va desde hace tres días.
Q. How would you describe the pain?	¿Cómo describiría el dolor?	¿Cómo es el dolor?
A. Well, it's an "aching pressure" that is across my chest. Sometimes it feels like a burning pain. Kind of like when you have real bad indigestion. Right now it feels like something is stuck in the middle of my chest.	Pues, es una presión dolorosa a lo largo de mi pecho. A veces lo siento como un dolor quemante. Como cuando uno tiene mucha indigestión. En este momento, siento como si tuviera algo atorado en la mitad del pecho.	Es una presión dolorosa a lo largo del pecho. A veces es como un dolor quemante (ardor). Como cuando uno tiene indigestión. Ahora siento como si tuviera algo atravesado en medio del pecho.
Q. Where is the pain located?	¿Dónde está localizado el dolor?	¿Dónde es el dolor?
A. The pain is throughout the center of my chest. There is really not one spot that I can pinpoint where this pain is.	El dolor es por todo el centro de mi pecho. Realmente no hay ningún lugar que yo pueda señalar dónde está el dolor.	El dolor está por todo el centro del pecho. No está sólo en un lugar.
Q. What makes it worse?	¿Qué empeora el dolor?	¿Qué lo hace peor?
A. The pain is worse when I drink or eat.	El dolor es peor cuando como o tomo algo.	Es peor cuando como o tomo algo.
Q. Is it worse with activity like running or walking?	¿Es peor con actividades como caminar o correr?	¿Es peor cuando camina o corre?
A. No, I run every morning and the pain is definitely not related to activity.	No, yo corro todas las mañanas y el dolor definitivamente no está asociado a la actividad.	No. Yo corro todos los días por la mañana y no siento dolor.
Q. Are there any foods or drinks which make the pain worse?	¿Hay algunas comidas o bebidas que empeoran el dolor?	¿Hay comidas o bebidas que lo hacen peor?
A. Cold foods are the worst, like ice cream. Also if I eat a lot at a time, it can sometimes bring on the pain.	Las comidas frías, como los helados (nieves), lo hacen peor. También a veces si como mucha comida a la vez, me puede comenzar el dolor.	Me duele cuando como comidas frías, como helados. También cuando como mucha cantidad.
Q. What makes it better?	¿Qué lo hace mejor (alivia)?	¿Qué le quita el dolor?
A. Nothing. The pain gets better on its own.	Nada. El dolor mejora por sí solo.	Nada. Se quita solo.
Q. Have you had this pain before?	¿Ha tenido este dolor anteriormente?	¿Ha tenido este dolor antes?
A. Yes. Over the past year I have had this pain, but it has gotten more frequent lately and more severe.	Sí. En el último año he tenido este dolor, pero se ha hecho más frecuente y más severo (fuerte) últimamente.	Sí. Lo he tenido todo el año, pero se ha hecho más fuerte y más frecuente.
Q. Does it come and go or is it constant?	¿Es constante o le viene y se le va?	¿Lo tiene todo el tiempo o le pega y se le quita?
A. It's a pain that comes and goes.	Es un dolor que viene y se va.	Me pega y se me quita.

	English	Spanish Formal	Spanish Informal Continued
Q.	Do you have burning in your chest at night or after eating a big meal?	¿Tiene quemazón (*ardor*) en el pecho por la noche o después de comer mucha comida?	¿Tiene quemazón de pecho en la noche o después de una comida muy grande?
A.	Yes, after I eat a large meal I do.	Sí, después de comer mucha comida.	Sí, después de comer mucho.
Q.	Does coffee or alcohol or chocolate cause the pain?	¿Le duele cuando toma café o licor o cuando come chocolate?	¿Le duele con café, licor o chocolate?
A.	It causes burning but not the pain I have now.	Me da quemazón pero no el dolor que siento ahora.	Me da ardor, pero no el dolor que tengo ahora.
Q.	Have you ever been treated with medicines to reduce the acid in your stomach?	¿Alguna vez le han dado medicinas para reducir el ácido del estómago?	¿Alguna vez le han dado tratamiento con antiácidos?
A.	No, I have not been given any medicines to reduce acid.	No, nunca me han dado medicinas para reducir la acidez.	No.
Q.	Are you having shortness of breath?	¿Tiene dificultad para respirar?	¿Siente que le falta el aire?
A.	No, my breathing is normal.	No, mi respiración es normal.	No.
Q.	Have you had any vomiting episodes?	¿Ha tenido algún episodio de vómito?	¿Ha vomitado?
A.	Yes, I have had several occasions in the past 3 days. I think I may have vomited 3 or 4 times right after eating.	Sí, he vomitado en varias ocasiones en los últimos tres días. Creo que vomité como tres o cuatro veces después de comer.	Sí, he vomitado varias veces en los últimos tres días. Vomité como tres o cuatro veces después de comer.
Q.	Do you have any abdominal pain?	¿Tiene dolor en el abdomen?	¿Tiene dolor de panza?
A.	No, I have not had any stomach pains.	No, no he tenido ningún dolor de estómago.	No.
Q.	Have you had any change in your bowel movements? Either constipation or diarrhea.	¿Ha tenido algún cambio a la hora de dar del cuerpo? Diarrea o estreñimiento (*constipación*).	¿Ha tenido diarrea o estreñimiento?
A.	No, everything is normal.	No, todo está normal.	No.
Q.	What medications are you taking?	¿Qué medicamentos está tomando?	¿Qué medicinas está tomando?
A.	None presently.	Ninguno, por el momento.	Ninguna.
Q.	Do you have any allergies to medications?	¿Tiene alguna alergia a los medicamentos?	¿Es alérgica a alguna medicina?
A.	No.	No.	No.
Q.	Do you have any medical illnesses?	¿Padece de alguna enfermedad?	¿Tiene alguna enfermedad?
A.	No, I am in good health except for the pain.	No, tengo buena salud excepto por el dolor.	No, sólo el dolor.
Q.	Do you smoke tobacco, drink alcohol, or use drugs such as cocaine?	¿Fuma cigarrillos, toma licor o usa drogas como cocaína?	¿Fuma, toma o usa drogas como cocaína?
A.	I don't smoke, and drink very rarely—at the most one beer on the weekends.	No fumo y tomo muy raramente, no más de una cerveza los fines de semana.	No fumo y tomo muy poco, sólo una cerveza los fines de semana.
Q.	Do you have any family history of diabetes, heart disease, gastrointestinal diseases, breast or cervical cancer or other illnesses that you know of?	Que usted sepa, ¿alguien en su familia padece de diabetes, enfermedades del corazón, enfermedades del aparato gastrointestinal, cáncer del busto, cáncer del cuello de la matriz o alguna otra enfermedad?	¿Alguien en su familia padece de alguna enfermedad seria como diabetes, del corazón, el estómago, los intestinos, cáncer del seno, cáncer del cerviz o alguna otra enfermedad?
A.	Yes, my sister has lupus.	Sí, mi hermana tiene lupus.	Mi hermana tiene lupus.

FOCUSED PHYSICAL EXAM

English	Spanish Formal	Spanish Informal
OK, I am going to perform a physical exam. Can you please change into this gown? I will need you to remove your shirt and bra so I can do a heart and lung exam. Your clothes below the waist can remain as is. I am going to step out while you change.	Está bien, le voy a hacer un examen físico. ¿Se puede poner esta bata, por favor? Necesito que se quite la blusa y el brasier (sostén) para poder hacerle un examen de corazón y pulmones. No tiene que quitarse la ropa debajo de la cintura. Voy a salir mientras se cambia.	Ahora le voy a hacer un examen. ¿Se puede poner esta bata? Tiene que quitarse la blusa y el brasier para examinarla. No tiene que quitarse la ropa debajo de la cintura. Voy a salir para que se desvista.
I need to listen to heart and lungs. Next I am going to do an abdominal exam. Sometimes chest pain can come from an intra-abdominal disease.	Necesito escuchar el corazón y los pulmones. Después le voy a examinar el abdomen. A veces el dolor de pecho es causado por una enfermedad abdominal.	Voy a escucharle el corazón y los pulmones. Después, a examinarle la panza. A veces el dolor de pecho es por una enfermedad en la panza.

PHYSICAL EXAM RESULTS

- **Vitals Signs**: Temp. 37.0° C, P 70, RR 14, BP 128/74.
- **General Appearance**: The patient appears to be uncomfortable but in no acute distress.
- **Lungs**: Clear to auscultation bilaterally.
- **Cardiovascular**: Regular rate, tachycardia. Normal S1 and S2. No S3 or S4 present. No murmurs, gallops, clicks, rub. No JVD present.
- **Abdomen**: Soft, flat, nontender, nondistended, no evidence of organomegaly, no masses, bowel sounds are normal.
- **Musculoskeletal**: no pain with chest palpation at costochondral joints or ribs.

DIFFERENTIAL DIAGNOSIS

- Non-cardiac, non-pulmonary origin of chest pain
- Esophageal disease: reflux, spasm
- Intra-abdominal pathology: biliary colic

This differential is quite different than the above cases. This is a young woman in good health who runs daily and does not smoke or use recreational drugs such as cocaine. The description of the pain and precipitating factors point to a noncardiac origin of the pain. Of note in the history is the complaint of burning in the retrosternal area, indicative of acid reflux disease. Reflux, while usually associated with this symptom, may also present less frequently with chest pain due to hypersensitivity of the esophageal mucosa to acid. Things that increase acid reflux from the stomach to the esophagus include alcohol, chocolate, fatty foods, caffeine and smoking, all factors that reduce the pressure in the lower esophageal sphincter (LES), a high pressure zone that inhibits acid from traveling from the stomach to the esophagus. Although this is the case in our patient, the precipitating factors such as cold liquid or food has no effect on reflux but is associated with esophageal spasm. Also, the transitory complaint of a sensation that "there is something stuck" is typical of spasm, which can cause a temporary obstruction. Often, reflux and esophageal spasm may present similarly, and other tests are needed to differentiate the two. Gallbladder disease, cholecystitis, typically presents with right upper quadrant pain but may occasionally present with chest pain. Especially in a young woman like this, it is not uncommon to see chest pain as a manifestation of biliary colic. The fact that she has no pulmonary complaints rules out a pulmonary etiology. Finally, there is no chest wall tenderness, ruling out costochondritis or rib fracture. The definitive workup can be done on an outpatient basis since there is no evidence of a life-threatening problem. To alleviate the symptoms of spasm, a calcium channel blocker such as diltiazem or nifedipine is utilized, while at the same time a proton pump inhibitor can be used to reduce acid secretion in the stomach and improve the symptoms of reflux. Although this is kind of a "shotgun approach" (i.e., treating disease without a definite diagnosis), that is what we do in clinical practice. You don't want your patient to continue hurting while she waits sometimes weeks or months for her definitive tests. The tests that will confirm her diagnosis of esophageal spasm include an upper gastrointestinal series, where the patient is given barium to swallow and an x-ray outlines the esophagus, demonstrating areas of spasm (Fig. 2-9). Intra-luminal pressure studies, esophageal manometry, of the esophagus will demonstrate uncoordinated peristaltic contractions.

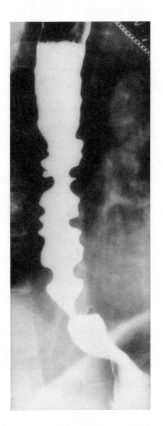

Figure 2-9. UGI series demonstrating spasm of the esophagus (nutmeg esophagus). (From Townsend C: *Sabiston Textbook of Surgery*, ed 17. Philadelphia, WB Saunders, 2004.)

DISCUSSION OF MANAGEMENT WITH THE PATIENT

English	Spanish Formal	Spanish Informal
Ms. Duarte, your history and physical exam point towards the esophagus—the tube connecting the mouth and stomach—as the cause of your pain. If the muscles of the esophagus spasm or too much acid goes from the stomach to the esophagus, severe chest pain can result. I will give you a prescription for two medicines, one to reduce the acid in the stomach and the other to relax the muscles of the esophagus. I am going to order a test where you swallow a material called barium. It is a white liquid that will outline the esophagus and may give us the diagnosis of spasm. I would like to see you back in a week to see if there is improvement in your symptoms. If the pain continues tomorrow, please call me. Do you have any questions?	Sra. Duarte, su historia y examen físico apuntan hacia el esófago, o sea, el tubo que conecta la boca con el estómago, como la causa de su dolor. Cuando los músculos del esófago sufren un espasmo o una gran cantidad de ácido va del estómago al esófago, se presenta un dolor severo. Le voy a dar una receta para dos medicinas. Una para reducir el ácido en el estómago y la otra para relajar los músculos del esófago. Voy a ordenar un examen en el que tiene que tragarse una sustancia que se llama bario. Es un líquido blanco que nos permite ver el contorno del esófago y nos puede ayudar a hacer el diagnóstico de espasmo. Me gustaría verla otra vez en una semana para ver si los síntomas han mejorado. Por favor, llámeme si el dolor continúa mañana. ¿Tiene alguna pregunta?	Sra. Duarte, todo parece indicar que el dolor que siente es por un problema del esófago, que es el tubo que conecta la boca con el estómago. Cuando hay un espasmo de los músculos del esófago o cuando ácido del estómago se va para el esófago, se presenta un dolor fuerte. Le voy a recetar una medicina para disminuir el ácido del estómago y otra para relajar los músculos del esófago. También voy a pedir un examen en el que tiene que tragarse una sustancia blanca que se llama bario, y que sirve para hacer el diagnóstico de espasmos. Quiero verla otra vez la próxima semana para ver si ha mejorado. Llámeme si sigue con dolor. ¿Tiene alguna pregunta?

PATHOPHYSIOLOGY

Esophageal spasms are a common disorder that present with clinical symptoms of chest pain. The spasms are a direct result of non-peristaltic contractions. These contractions are of long duration and amplitude. Histopathological studies show prominent degeneration of nerve processes. These spasms may represent cholinergic or myogenic hypersensitivity. Anticholinergics provide limited resolution. Smooth muscle relaxants such as nitroglycerin or longer acting agents such as isosorbide dinitrate and nifedipine are first-line treatment choices.

CASE 4: PULMONARY EMBOLUS

CHIEF COMPLAINT

Mrs. Gallegos is a 29-year-old who presents with acute onset of shortness of breath.

Vital signs: BP 124/78, P 110, RR 32/min.

As you walk into the room, she is agitated and in moderate respiratory distress with obvious tachypnea. In this situation, you want to listen to the lung fields prior to anything else. Remember Airway, Breathing, and Circulation: the ABCs.

HISTORY

	English	Spanish Formal	Spanish Informal
Q.	Hi, Mrs. Gallegos, I am Dr. Austin, are you having a lot of trouble breathing?	Hola, Sra. Gallegos, soy el Dr. Austin. ¿Tiene mucha dificultad para respirar?	Sra. Gallegos, soy el Dr. Austin. ¿Le cuesta mucho respirar?
A.	Yes, doctor, I can't catch my breath.	Sí, doctor, no puedo respirar.	Sí, doctor, me cuesta respirar.
Q.	We are going to put some oxygen on to ease your breathing and we are going to put a pulse oximeter to measure the oxygen in your blood. I also need to listen to your lungs.	Le vamos a poner algo de oxígeno para que pueda respirar mejor y vamos a ponerle un oxímetro para medir el nivel de oxígeno en su sangre. También necesito escucharle los pulmones.	Vamos a darle oxígeno para que pueda respirar mejor y a ponerle un oxímetro para medirle el oxígeno en la sangre. También tengo que oírle los pulmones.
	Your lungs are clear.	Sus pulmones no tienen secreciones.	Sus pulmones están bien.

The fact that the patient can talk to you coherently usually means A is okay. Good breath sounds bilaterally and clear lung fields take care of B.

Blood pressure is good; C is stable although it is wise to establish an intravenous line in case our patient deteriorates.

Immediately place the patient on oxygen and see if there is improvement. Also place a pulse oximeter on the patient to measure blood oxygen saturation transcutaneously.

	English	Spanish Formal	Spanish Informal
Q.	Are you feeling better?	¿Se siente mejor?	¿Está mejor?
A.	I am breathing easier but still not normal.	Estoy respirando con menos dificultad pero todavía no es normal.	Estoy respirando mejor. Todavía no es normal.

Pulse oximeter reads 88% on 40% fraction of inspired oxygen (FIO_2).

The pulse oximeter reads the saturation of hemoglobin with oxygen. Normally, on room air this should be over 90%. On a 40% inspired oxygen normally this should be above 95%. The fact that our patient is only 88% tells us that there is an intra-pulmonic "shunt." In other words, blood is going to the lung but not being oxygenated and returning to the left atrium unoxygenated.

The fact that she is more stable now allows us to proceed with the focused history and physical exam. We still need to move quickly, however.

	English	Spanish Formal	Spanish Informal
Q.	What brings you to see us today, Mrs. Gallegos?	¿Por qué viene a vernos hoy, Sra. Gallegos?	¿Por qué vino hoy, Sra. Gallegos?
A.	I can't catch my breath.	No puedo respirar.	Me cuesta respirar.
Q.	How old are you, Mrs. Gallegos?	¿Qué edad tiene, Sra. Gallegos?	¿Qué edad tiene?
A.	I am 29 years old.	Tengo veintinueve años.	Veintinueve años.

	English	Spanish Formal	Spanish Informal
Q.	How long ago did you become short of breath?	¿Hace cuánto comenzó a tener dificultad para respirar?	¿Desde cuándo le cuesta respirar?
A.	It started suddenly about an hour ago.	Me comenzó súbitamente hace como una hora.	Me comenzó de pronto, hace una hora.
Q.	Has it gotten worse?	¿Ha empeorado?	¿Está peor ahora?
A.	Yes. With the oxygen, though, I feel a lot better.	Sí. Pero con el oxígeno ahora me siento mucho mejor.	Sí. Pero me siento mejor con el oxígeno ahora.
Q.	Have you had any chest pain?	¿Ha tenido dolor de pecho?	¿Ha tenido dolor de pecho?
A.	Yes. My chest hurts when I take a deep breath in.	Sí. Me duele el pecho cuando respiro profundo.	Sí. Me duele cuando respiro fuerte (*recio*).
Q.	On a scale of 1 to 10, 10 being the worst pain you have ever had, how would you rate the pain?	En una escala de uno a diez, donde diez es el peor dolor que usted ha tenido en su vida, ¿cómo catalogaría (*clasificaría*) este dolor?	Si tuviera que clasificar este dolor de uno a diez, y diez fuera el peor dolor que usted ha tenido en su vida, ¿cómo diría usted que es este dolor?
A.	About a 5.	Alrededor de cinco.	Como un. . . cinco.
Q.	Is it sharp or dull?	¿Es un dolor agudo (*punzante*) o sordo?	¿Es un dolor sordo o como una punzada (*puñalada*)?
A.	It is sharp.	Es punzante (*agudo*).	Como una punzada.
Q.	Does it come and go?	¿Viene y se va?	¿Le pega y se le quita?
A.	It is constant.	Es constante.	Lo tengo todo el tiempo (*no se me quita*).
Q.	What makes it worse or better?	¿Qué lo hace mejor o peor?	¿Qué lo mejora y qué lo empeora?
A.	When I take a deep breath in it hurts, but if I breathe shallow, it hurts a lot less.	Cuando respiro profundamente me duele, pero si respiro superficialmente me duele mucho menos.	Me duele cuando respiro recio (*fuerte*). Me duele menos cuando respiro quedito (*superficialmente*).
Q.	Have you had a fever or a cough?	¿Ha tenido fiebre o tos?	¿Ha tenido calentura o tos?
A.	No, I have had no fever or cough.	No, no he tenido calentura ni tos.	No.
Q.	Have you had chest pain like this before?	¿Ha tenido un dolor de pecho como este anteriormente?	¿Ha tenido un dolor como este antes?
A.	No, I have never had this kind of pain before.	No, nunca he tenido este tipo de dolor antes.	No, nunca.
Q.	Have you had shortness of breath like this before?	¿Ha tenido dificultad para respirar anteriormente?	¿Ha tenido falta de aire antes?
A.	No, not like this.	No, así como esto, no.	No.
Q.	Do you have any lung diseases like asthma?	¿Tiene alguna enfermedad de los pulmones, como asma?	¿Padece de los pulmones? ¿Tiene asma?
A.	When I was little, they thought I might have had asthma, but I haven't had problems as an adult.	Cuando era pequeña (*niña, chica*) pensaba que podía padecer de asma, pero no he tenido problemas de adulta (*grande*).	Cuando chica, pensaba que iba a padecer de asma, pero no he vuelto a tener problemas.
Q.	Do you have any heart problems?	¿Tiene problemas del corazón?	¿Padece del corazón?
A.	I have no heart problems.	No tengo problemas del corazón.	No.

	English	Spanish Formal	Spanish Informal Continued
Q.	Can you run or walk a mile without chest pain or shortness of breath?	¿Puede caminar o correr una milla sin dolor de pecho o dificultad para respirar?	¿Puede caminar o correr una milla sin tener dolor de pecho o falta de aire?
A.	Yes. I workout three to four times a week.	Sí, hago ejercicio tres o cuatro veces a la semana.	Sí, hago ejercicio regularmente.
Q.	Are you on any medications?	¿Esta tomando algún medicamento?	¿Toma alguna medicina?
A.	Yes. I take birth control pills.	Sí. Tomo pastillas anticonceptivas.	Sí. Pastillas para evitar el embarazo.
Q.	Do you smoke tobacco or have you ever smoked?	¿Fuma cigarrillos o ha fumado alguna vez?	¿Alguna vez ha fumado cigarrillos?
A.	I have never smoked.	Nunca he fumado.	No.
Q.	Have you recently been on any long trips where you had to sit for a long time?	Recientemente, ¿ha hecho algún viaje largo en el que tuvo que estar sentada por mucho tiempo?	¿Ha hecho algún viaje largo en el que tuvo que estar sentada por mucho tiempo?
A.	No, I haven't traveled recently.	No, no he viajado recientemente.	Tampoco.
Q.	Have you had surgery in the past?	¿Ha tenido alguna cirugía en el pasado?	¿Alguna vez la han operado?
A.	Yes. I had my gallbladder removed two months ago.	Sí. Me quitaron la vesícula biliar hace dos meses.	Me operaron de la vesícula hace un par de meses.
Q.	Have you had any leg swelling in the past?	¿Alguna vez se le han hinchado (inflamado) los pies?	¿Ha tenido hinchazón de los pies alguna vez?
A.	No. I have not noticed any swelling of my legs.	No. No he notado ninguna inflamación de mis piernas.	No.
Q.	Do you have any allergies to medications?	¿Es alérgica a algún medicamento?	¿Padece de alergia a alguna medicina?
A.	No. I have no allergies.	No. No padezco de alergias.	No.

PHYSICAL EXAM

Vital signs: BP 122/78, P 100, RR 22, Temp. 37.6° C; Pulse orimeter 88% on 40% FIO_2 by Face Mask.

- **General Appearance**: The patient is much more comfortable than when she first presented but still tachypnic.
- **Chest**: Lungs clear to auscultation, good breath sounds bilaterally, no rales or rhonchi are present.
- **Heart**: Sinus tachycardia is present, normal S1 and S2, no S3 or S4, no murmurs are heard. No JVD is present.
- **Abdominal Exam**: Unremarkable.
- **Lower Extremities**: No swelling present.

DIFFERENTIAL DIAGNOSIS

The history and physical exam points to a pulmonary source. Our patient is young with a main complaint of shortness of breath and chest pain. The fact that her lungs are clear rules out a pneumothorax, which would produce decreased breath sounds on the side of the lesion due to collapse of the lung by air filling the ipsilateral pleural space. Pneumonia is ruled out for the same reason as well as the absence of fever and cough. A real red flag is the use of birth control pills, which predispose to deep vein thrombosis and subsequent pulmonary embolus. Also, the history of recent surgery predisposes to the development of deep vein thrombosis. This can be a life-threatening condition. One needs to make a definitive diagnosis and then treat with anticoagulants so no further emboli break off to the lung. The classic triad of pulmonary embolus is tachypnea, tachycardia, and chest pain. Typically, the lungs are clear since there is in most cases no effect on aeration of the alveoli. Hypoxemia is almost always present due to the shunt in the lung. Chest x-ray is ordered to rule out any disease such as pneumonia but also to see if there is a pulmonary infarct, which is unusual but may be seen with a large pulmonary embolus. Typically, the chest x-ray is normal. A blood gas is also ordered to assess the degree of hypoxemia.

DISCUSSION OF MANAGEMENT WITH THE PATIENT

	English	Spanish Formal	Spanish Informal
Q.	Mrs. Gallegos, we are going to order some blood tests, an x-ray of the chest, and an ECG. I think you have a pulmonary embolus, which is a clot in the vessels going to the lungs. Usually they come from a clot in the veins of the legs or pelvis. These tests will help confirm the diagnosis. If that is what you have, then we will give you a blood thinner, heparin, through the vein to prevent any other clot from going to the lung. We will also order a lung scan, which is a test that will show us if a clot has gone to the lung. You will need to be admitted to the hospital for treatment. Do you have any questions?	Sra. Gallegos, vamos a ordenar unos exámenes de sangre, una radiografía de tórax y un ECG. Yo pienso que usted tiene una embolia pulmonar, que es un coágulo en los vasos sanguíneos que van para los pulmones. Generalmente, son coágulos que se forman en las venas de las piernas o de la cadera. Estas pruebas nos ayudarán a confirmar el diagnóstico. Si eso es lo que tiene, entonces le vamos a dar una medicina que se llama heparina para "adelgazar" la sangre (*un anticoagulante*). La heparina se pone por la vena para prevenir que otros coágulos se vayan a los pulmones. También vamos a ordenar una tomografía de pulmón, que es una prueba para ver si algún coágulo se ha ido al pulmón. La vamos a tener que internar en el hospital para darle tratamiento. ¿Tiene alguna pregunta?	Sra. Gallegos, le vamos a hacer unas pruebas de sangre, una radiografía del pecho, un ECG. Pienso que tiene una embolia pulmonar, que es un coágulo en los vasos que van a los pulmones. Usualmente, son coágulos que se forman en las venas de las piernas o de la cadera. Las pruebas nos ayudarán a confirmar el diagnóstico. Si eso es lo que tiene, entonces le vamos a dar heparina, una medicina para "adelgazar" la sangre. La heparina se pone por la vena para evitar que otros coágulos se vayan a los pulmones. También le vamos a hacer una tomografía del pulmón, una prueba para ver si algún coágulo se ha ido al pulmón. La vamos a internar en el hospital para darle tratamiento. ¿Tiene preguntas?
A.	Is it serious? Will I be in the hospital a long time?	¿Es un problema serio? ¿Voy a estar en el hospital por mucho tiempo?	¿Es una cosa grave? ¿Cuánto voy a estar en el hospital?
Q.	Yes, but if we treat it early like we are doing, we will prevent any further clot from going to the lung. The clot that is already there will slowly dissolve and disappear, and you will breathe normal following that. Most people are in the hospital for about a week or a little less. Once the blood is thinned by the heparin, they will give you pills, Coumadin, which you take by mouth. Once these thin the blood sufficiently, you can be discharged home.	Sí, pero si lo tratamos temprano como lo estamos haciendo, vamos a prevenir que más coágulos se vayan para los pulmones. El coágulo que ya está ahí se va a disolver lentamente y va a desaparecer, y usted va a poder respirar normalmente después de eso. La mayor parte de las personas están en el hospital por una semana o un poco menos. Una vez que la sangre esté "adelgazada" con la heparina, le van a dar pastillas de Coumadin para tomar por la boca. Una vez que estas pastillas le "adelgacen" la sangre lo suficiente, le daremos la salida.	Sí, pero si lo tratamos a tiempo, como ahora, vamos a evitar que más coágulos se vayan a los pulmones. El coágulo que ya está ahí se va a deshacer (*desbaratar*) y desaparecer, usted va a poder respirar bien después. Por lo general, las personas con esta enfermedad están en el hospital una semana o menos. Una vez que la sangre esté "adelgazada" con la heparina, le vamos a dar pastillas de Coumadin para tomar. Y una vez que estas pastillas estén trabajando, le vamos a dar la salida.

VOCABULARY

English	Español
Angina	Dolor de pecho, angina de pecho
Angiogram	Angiograma, angiografía, procedimiento para obtener una imagen del interior de los vasos sanguíneos
Aortic aneurysm	Aneurisma aórtico, debilidad en la pared de la aorta
Aortic dissection	Disección de la aorta
Aortic valve	Válvula aórtica
Bilateral pedal edema	Edema bipedal, inflamación o hinchazón de ambas piernas
Blockage	Obstrucción, bloqueo
Bra	Brasier, sostén, sujetador
Cardiac arrhythmias	Arritmia cardíaca, irregularidad de las contracciones del corazón
Cardiac catheterization	Cateterismo cardíaco, introducir un catéter por un vaso sanguíneo hasta llegar al corazón
Catheter	Catéter, sonda
Complete blood count	Hemograma completo, conteo de células de la sangre
Congestive heart failure	Insuficiencia cardíaca congestiva
Coronary arteries	Arterias coronarias
Coronary bypass	Desviación o derivación coronaria, una operación del corazón en la que se coloca un vaso sanguíneo como "puente" para permitir el paso de sangre alrededor de una zona obstruida
Costochondritis	Costocondritis, inflamación de la articulación de la costilla y el esternón
Cough	Tos
Chest CT	Tomografía computarizada del pecho (tórax)
Chest pain	Dolor de pecho
Chest wall contusion	Contusión en la pared costal, golpe en el pecho (en las costillas)
Chest x-ray	Radiografía de tórax, rayos X del pecho
Cholecystitis	Colecistitis, inflamación de la vesícula biliar
Choledocholithiasis	Coledocolitiasis, piedras o cálculos en la vesícula
Chronic bronchitis	Bronquitis crónica
Chronic obstructive pulmonary disease (COPD)	Enfermedad pulmonar obstructiva crónica (EPOC)
Deep vein thrombosis	Trombosis (coágulo) de las venas profundas
Dizzy	Mareado
Emergency department	Departamento de urgencias o de emergencias
Esophageal reflux	Reflujo esofágico, agruras, acidez, reflujo

English	Español
Esophageal spasm	Espasmo esofágico, contracción de los músculos del esófago
Esophagitis	Esofagitis, inflamación del esófago
Faint	Desmayo, desmayarse, perder la conciencia, perder el sentido
Heart	Corazón
Heart murmur	Soplo cardíaco, soplo del corazón
Herpes Zoster (Shingles)	Herpes Zoster, herpes
Hypertension	Hipertensión arterial, presión alta
Ischemia	Isquemia, falta de oxígeno en una parte del cuerpo (isquemia del corazón)
Lightheaded	Mareado, tener mareo, sentir como si se fuera a desmayar
Lower esophageal sphincter	Esfínter esofágico inferior
Mitral valve	Válvula mitral
Myocardial infarction	Infarto del miocardio, ataque del corazón
Nasal oxygen	Oxígeno por la nariz
Numbness	Entumecimiento, adormecimiento
Open heart surgery	Cirugía u operación de corazón abierto
Outpatient clinic	Clínica de consulta externa
Palpitations	Palpitaciones
Pancreatitis	Pancreatitis, inflamación del páncreas
Panic disorder	Trastorno de pánico, ataque de pánico
Peptic ulcer	Úlcera péptica, úlcera
Pericarditis	Pericarditis, inflamación de la cubierta (envoltura) del corazón
Peripheral vascular disease	Enfermedad vascular periférica, enfermedad de los vasos sanguíneos
Phlegm	Flemas, gargajos, esputos
Pleuritis	Pleuritis, inflamación de la cubierta (envoltura) del pulmón
Pneumonia	Neumonía, pulmonía
Pneumothorax	Neumotórax
Pulmonary embolism	Embolismo pulmonar, embolia del pulmón
Pulse oximeter	Oxímetro de pulso, oxímetro
Rales, crackles	Estertores crepitaciones
Rib fracture	Fractura costal, fractura o quebradura de la costilla
Rub	Frotar, rozar
Scapula, shoulder blade	Escápula, omóplato
Sharp, stabbing pain	Dolor agudo, punzante, como una puñalada
Shortness of breath	Dificultad para respirar, falta de aire, ahogo

English	Español	Continued
Squeezing pain	Dolor opresivo, apretazón, como que me apretaran	
Sterno-clavicular arthritis	Artritis (inflamación) de la articulación de la clavícula y el esternón	
Sternum	Esternón, hueso del pecho	
Swelling	Inflamación, hinchazón	
Tightness	Apretazón	
Tingling	Hormigueo	
Trauma	Trauma, golpe	
Ventricular fibrillation	Fibrilación ventricular, contracciones de los ventrículos del corazón	
Wheezing	Sibilancia, ruido sibilante, silbido agudo	

GRAMMATICAL TIPS

PRESENT SUBJUNCTIVE

It is formed by taking the *yo* person in the present tense and adding the endings to the conjugation.

For the present subjunctive, the endings are as follows:

Verb subject	*Hablar* = to speak	*Comer* = to eat	*Vivir* = to live
I = *Yo*	Habl – **e**	Com – **a**	Viv – **a**
You (informal) = *Tú*	Habl – **es**	Com – **as**	Viv – **as**
He/She/You (formal) = *Él, Ella, Usted*	Habl – **e**	Com – **a**	Viv – **a**
We = *Nosotros, Nosotras*	Habl – **emos**	Com – **amos**	Viv – **amos**
You (plural)/They = *Ustedes, Ellos, Ellas*	Habl – **en**	Com – **an**	Viv – **an**

Notice that the present subjunctive endings are transposed to the endings in the present tense and the only difference is the *yo* conjugation.

Uses of the Subjunctive
It is a subjective mood that applies to different tenses. Whenever something is uncertain, those verbs should trigger the subjunctive.

Verbs that trigger the subjunctive are verbs to express wanting, requesting, emotion, doubting, denial, impersonal expressions, negation, giving advice.

The subjunctive is formed with two subjects and a word (*que*) that unites both sentences, and the second verb is in the subjunctive because the first verb triggers it.

Look at the following example:

Quiero que tú vengas a mi consultorio.

The first sentence is *quiero* and what makes that subjunctive is the wanting verb conjugated in the present indicative tense. The *que* unites both sentences. The second sentence *tú vengas a mi consultorio* is the subjunctive clause because the result of the wanting is subjective: Yes, I do want you to come but I am uncertain as to whether you will come or not.

Remember that if the first sentence implies wanting, requesting, emotion, doubting, denial, impersonal expressions, negation, or giving advice, then the subjunctive is triggered. The speaker also decides whether or not he or she will use the subjunctive mood depending upon uncertainty.

EXERCISE

Please choose from the options below if the sentence is certain or uncertain. If it is uncertain, it will be subjunctive; if certain, it will be indicative. Then fill in the blanks appropriately, conjugating the verbs in the correct form: present indicative or subjunctive. (¡ojo!) *Ojalá* has its root in Arabic and it is used in Spanish. It means "God grant" or "God willing."

¿Subjuntivo o Indicativo?

Subj. Ind. 1. La enfermera quiere que nosotros _____ (hablar) con el doctor.

Subj. Ind. 2. Ojalá que el examen de sangre no _____ (resultar) positivo.

Subj. Ind. 3. La niña desea que sus abuelos no la _____ (llevar) al dentista.

Subj. Ind. 4. Yo te recomiendo que tú _____ (hacer) una cita.

Subj. Ind. 5. Concepción no duda de que ellas _____ (dejar) de fumar.

Subj. Ind. 6. Ellos quieren que yo _____ (ir) al hospital.

Subj. Ind. 7. Ernesto no cree que sus hijos _____ (estar) enfermos.

Subj. Ind. 8. Es cierto que hoy _____ (ser) el día de tu operación.

Subj. Ind. 9. Esperanza sugiere que tú no le _____ (decir) la verdad.

Subj. Ind. 10. Siempre es mejor que la gente _____ (expresar) sus problemas de salud.

Notice that there are very few irregular verbs compared to the present tense or *pretérito*. Here is a list of 6 of them:

Dar = to give	Estar = to be	Haber = to have (aux.)	Ir = to go	Saber = to know	Ser = to be
Dé	Esté	Haya	Vaya	Sepa	Sea
Des	Estés	Hayas	Vayas	Sepas	Seas
Dé	Esté	Haya	Vaya	Sepa	Sea
Demos	Estemos	Hayamos	Vayamos	Sepamos	Seamos
Deis	Estéis	Hayáis	Vayáis	Sepáis	Seáis
Den	Estén	Hayan	Vayan	Sepan	Sean

There are verbs that change their spelling also because of phonetic reasons.

Commands Are Also Formed With the Subjunctive

Affirmative and negative commands are formed with the subjunctive mood, with the exception of the *tú* affirmative command.

For example: The verbs *hablar, comer,* and *vivir* and their respective affirmative and negative commands are included in the following set. In the negative form, you will need to add a *no* in front of the verb.

	Hablar	Comer	Vivir
Tú negative command	No hables	No comas	No vivas
Él, Ellas, and *Usted*	Hable	Coma	Viva
Nosotros	Hablemos	Comamos	Vivamos
Ustedes, Ellos, Ellas	Hablen	Coman	Vivan

The exception is the affirmative *tú* command, which is formed by using the third person singular (*él, ella, usted* form) of the present tense.
Habla = speak (you); *Come* = eat (you); *Vive* = live (you)

There are eight irregular *tú* commands. Here is the list. Notice that for the four from the first column, you only take the ending away and you are left with the *tú* command.

Irregular *tú* Affirmative Commands
Salir = Sal
Tener = Ten
Venir = Ven
Poner = Pon
Ir = Ve
Hacer = Haz
Decir = Di
Ser = Sé

It is helpful to look at the dialogues and try to identify the subjunctive and the commands within the conversations.

CULTURAL TIPS: EMPACHO

Within the cultural approach comes the understanding that many patients coming from Spanish-speaking countries who have a traditional mindset about medicine also feel that their condition or illness influences what they do to find relief. Some Spanish-speaking patients with abdominal pain, particularly those who come from underserved communities, may believe that they have a condition called *empacho*.

Empacho is a non-medical term for a type of indigestion that affects the population in general. The most common symptoms for empacho are abdominal pain, indigestion, bloating, lack of appetite, feeling that there is something stuck to the esophagus, fever, vomiting, sourness, and diarrhea. It is believed that being forced to eating against one's will causes this condition, or that eating dough or uncooked foods will cause it too. Others believe that it is the result of eating excessive amounts of one type of food such as cheese, eggs, or *chicharrones* (fried pork skin). Whatever the cause, the belief is that eating these foods causes an accumulation of poorly digested food in the intestines or the esophagus. Some people argue that the food actually gets stuck to the walls of the intestine.

Some actions to resolve an empacho include drinking *té de manzanilla* (chamomile tea) or *yerbabuena* (mint tea). Some people go to *curanderos/as* or *yerberos/as,* who sometimes pinch and pull at their abdomen to help "dislodge" the food, or massage the stomach in a down motion while the patient is fasting. Such massage is done with a certain oil.

During the focused history, health professionals should explore patients' understanding of their illness and its causes. Questions such as these should be asked: What do you believe caused your disease? What do you call such disease, and describe it to me, Are you taking home remedies? What are the results of such remedies? Have you consulted with a physician in Mexico or a *curandero* before coming to see me? When you ask your patients if they have used traditional medicines to cure themselves and the answer is "yes, but it has not worked," you can offer them your treatment and encourage them to take it without diminishing or dismissing the traditional healer or curandero who first prescribed them treatment. It is important that the patient feels that you respect his or her beliefs and don't consider him or her backward for believing in traditional healers.

3 Pediatric Emergencies

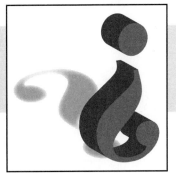

INTRODUCTION

Pediatric emergencies cover a wide range of disease states. In this chapter, we will cover common infectious diseases seen in this group of patients. These constitute the majority of pediatric emergencies seen by the clinician. Certain anatomic and immunologic differences exist between the adult and the child, predisposing the latter to certain infectious diseases. Often fever is the most common complaint in children presenting with infection. The key is to decide whether this is a serious problem such as meningitis—a serious infection of the spinal canal that will require admission to the hospital along with careful monitoring and treatment with antibiotics—or a more mild disease such as a viral upper respiratory infection that will get better without treatment. The degree of fever is often a poor indicator of the severity of infection. It is not uncommon to see a child with a viral upper respiratory infection with fever to 39 °C and a child with septicemia, a life-threatening blood-borne infection, with a temperature below normal range. The cases that are presented in this chapter will demonstrate how we differentiate the severely ill child from the child suffering from the common diseases seen in this age range that may require no treatment at all.

CASE 1: OTITIS MEDIA

CHIEF COMPLAINT

A two-year-old girl presents to Urgent Care with a chief complaint of fever, congestion, and a cough.

HISTORY

English	Spanish Formal	Spanish Informal
Hello, Ms. Rivas, my name is Carla Jones. I am a third year medical student working with Dr. Garza and I will be asking you and your daughter some questions.	Hola, señora Rivas, mi nombre es Carlos Jones. Soy estudiante de medicina de tercer año. Trabajo con el Dr. Garza y les voy a hacer unas preguntas a usted y a su hija.	Hola, señora Rivas, soy Carlos Jones, estudiante de medicina de tercer año. Trabajo con el Dr. Garza y le voy a hacer unas preguntas.
Q. How old is Denise?	¿Qué edad tiene Denise?	¿Cuántos años tiene Denise?
A. Two years old.	Dos años.	Dos.
Q. What brings you to see us today?	¿Por qué viene a vernos hoy?	¿Por qué vino?
A. My daughter has a fever.	Mi hija tiene fiebre.	La niña está con calentura.
Q. How long has she had a fever and how high has it gotten?	¿Desde cuándo ha tenido fiebre y qué tan alto le ha subido?	¿Cuándo le comenzó? ¿Cuánto ha tenido?
A. She has had a fever since two days ago. I don't have a thermometer, but she has felt real hot and has been crying all the time.	Ha tenido fiebre desde hace dos días. No tengo termómetro, pero la he sentido muy caliente y ha estado llorando todo el tiempo.	Empezó hace dos días. No tengo termómetro, pero ha estado muy caliente y llorando mucho.
Q. Have you given her any medicine for the temperature, and if so, how often?	¿Le ha dado alguna medicina para la fiebre? Y de ser así, ¿con qué frecuencia?	¿Le ha dado algo para la calentura? ¿Cuántas veces al día?
A. Yes, I have been giving her Tylenol every six hours. It takes the fever down but then it goes up a few hours later.	Sí, le he estado dando Tylenol cada seis horas. Le baja la fiebre pero le sube otra vez unas horas después.	Le estoy dando Tylenol cada seis horas, pero la calentura vuelve a subir al rato.
Q. Has she had any vomiting or diarrhea?	¿Ha tenido vómitos o diarrea?	¿Ha vomitado? ¿Ha tenido diarrea?
A. She has not vomited nor had diarrhea.	No ha vomitado ni tenido diarrea.	No.
Q. Is she taking liquids in well and eating well?	¿Está tomado líquidos bien y comiendo bien?	¿Ha comido? ¿Ha tomado agua o refrescos?
A. She isn't eating well but she is drinking liquids well.	No está comiendo bien pero está tomando líquidos sin dificultad.	No ha comido casi nada pero está tomando aguas frescas.
Q. Is she active and playful or is she irritable and cranky?	¿Está activa y jugando o irritable y de mal humor *(enojada, enfadada)*?	¿Está jugando bien o está enfadada y de mal humor?
A. She is cranky and cries most of the time. She isn't sleeping at all.	Está de mal humor y llora casi todo el tiempo. No está durmiendo nada.	Está muy llorona y de malhumor. Y no duerme nada.
Q. Is she urinating about the same as before or do you have to change her diapers less frequently?	¿Está orinando casi igual que antes o tiene que cambiarle los pañales con menos frecuencia?	¿Está orinando normal? ¿Está usando menos pañales?
A. No, about the same as before.	No, igual que antes.	Igual que antes.
Q. Has she been grabbing or pulling at her ears?	¿Se ha estado tocando o halando las orejas?	¿Se está halando las orejas?
A. Yes, she has been pulling at her left ear and crying.	Sí, ha estado llorando y halándose la oreja izquierda.	Sí, se hala la oreja izquierda y llora.
Q. Has she had a cough or runny nose?	¿Ha tenido tos o mocos por la nariz *(suelta de la nariz)*?	¿Ha estado tosiendo o mormada?
A. Yes, she has been very congested and has a cough.	Sí, ha estado muy constipada *(mormada, con mucha congestión)* y tiene tos.	Ha estado muy mormada y tiene tos.

	English	Spanish Formal	Spanish Informal
Q.	Has she ever had an ear infection before?	¿Alguna vez ha tenido una infección del oído?	¿Ha tenido infección de oído?
A.	No, she has been very healthy up to now.	No, hasta ahora siempre ha sido muy saludable.	No.
Q.	Do think she has had any problems hearing you during her illness?	¿Usted piensa que ella ha tenido dificultad para escuchar?	¿Tiene problemas para oír?
A.	Yes, at times I talk to her and she acts as if she isn't listening.	Sí, a veces le hablo y parece que no me estuviera escuchando.	Sí, a veces parece que no me escucha.
Q.	Is there anyone in the home with any infection?	¿Hay alguien en su casa con alguna infección?	¿Alguien más en la casa está enfermo?
A.	Her five-year-old brother has a cold but he is getting better.	El hermanito de cinco años está resfriado pero está mejorando.	El hermano está resfriado también, pero ahora está mejor.
Q.	Does your daughter have any history of bronchitis, recurrent diarrhea, strep throat, or urinary tract infections?	¿Alguna vez su hija ha tenido bronquitis, diarrea (recurrente), infección de la garganta o infección de las vías urinarias?	¿Alguna vez ha padecido de los bronquios, la garganta, mal de orín o diarrea?
A.	No.	No.	No.
Q.	Are her immunizations up to date?	¿Está al día con las vacunas?	¿Tiene todas las vacunas?
A.	Yes, she was immunized last month.	Sí, le pusieron una vacuna el mes pasado.	Sí, la última se la pusieron hace un mes.

The immediate goal in evaluating the pediatric patient with fever is to decide if the infectious process is a life-threatening condition. Certain diseases such as meningitis need to be diagnosed and treated as quickly as possible. The initial history is a crucial part of this decision-making. Infants with meningitis or sepsis (overwhelming infection) stop eating; they lose their appetite. They also stop taking in fluids because they are so weak from the infection. The parent will also note that the infant is listless, lethargic, and often the crying of the baby is weak or has ceased completely. This is a grave sign. It is ironic that when we evaluate a febrile infant in the emergency room who has a strong cry and tears we are relieved, versus a baby who presents with fever and who is lethargic and quiet.

The infant just discussed is taking in fluids and is crying. Of note, the baby is urinating (as noted by the changing of diapers), a sign of adequate hydration status. Another good sign of adequate hydration is the presence of tears. In an infant who is not taking in an adequate quantity of fluids due to severe infection or whose fluid losses are greater than normal—as seen in gastroenteritis (with its accompanying diarrhea)—dehydration develops rapidly. Especially in infants under one year of age, the concentrating ability of the kidney may be poorly developed, setting the stage for intravascular volume depletion and hypovolemia. In addition, the large surface area in comparison to weight in the infant makes evaporative loss, when fever is present, a significant problem. Of note is the fact that the infant is pulling at her ears, a giveaway to the diagnosis of otitis media, an infection of the middle ear. Often this is accompanied by an upper respiratory infection. In the infant, the Eustachian tube is much more horizontal than in the adult (Fig. 3-1). This horizontal position inhibits drainage of the middle ear, thus predisposing to overgrowth of bacteria and infection. The high frequency of upper respiratory

Figure 3-1. Anatomy of the eustachian tube. Note the horizontal position of the tube in the infant and the vertical position in the adult. (Modified from Bluestone CD, Klein JO: *Pediatric Otolaryngology*. Philadelphia, WB Saunders, 1996.)

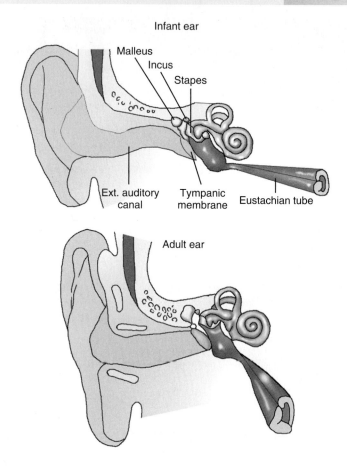

Infant ear

Malleus
Incus
Stapes
Ext. auditory canal
Tympanic membrane
Eustachian tube

Adult ear

infections in the pediatric patient also predisposes to blockage of the Eustachian tube. As seen in Figure 3-1, the Eustachian tube drains into the pharynx, where the adenoids are located. The adenoids are a mass of lymphatic tissues that swells with any upper respiratory infection, increasing the risk of otitis media by obstructing the tube. Thus, the incidence of otitis media is highest in the younger child, especially under the age of 10.

The next step is the physical exam.

THE PHYSICAL EXAM

	English	Spanish Formal	Spanish Informal
Q.	Ms. Rivas, I am going to perform the physical exam. Can you hold Denise while I perform the initial physical exam? During the exam of the throat and ears, the nurse will assist me (we always leave the most traumatic exam for last, i.e., the throat and ears due to the fact that usually the infant will cry after these two exams, which would make listening to the heart and lungs very difficult).	Sra. Rivas, voy a hacer el examen físico. ¿Puede sostener a Denise mientras comienzo a examinarla? La enfermera me va a ayudar mientras examino la garganta y los oídos (siempre dejamos el examen más traumático para el final, por ejemplo los oídos y la garganta, porque por lo general el niño llorará después de estos dos exámenes, haciendo más difícil escuchar el corazón y los pulmones).	Sra. Rivas, voy a examinar a Denise. ¿Puede sostenerla? La enfermera me va a ayudar mientras examino la garganta y los oídos.
A.	Of course.	Claro que sí.	Está bien.

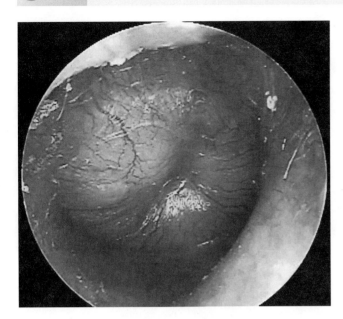

Figure 3-2. Inflammation of the tympanic membranes in a child with acute otitis media. (From Behrman R, Kliegman R, Jenson H: *Nelson Textbook of Pediatrics*, ed 17. Philadelphia, Saunders, 2004.)

The physical exam reveals a crying, irritable infant. Good tear formation is noted. Temperature is 38.2° C, respiratory rate 24, and pulse 120. Inflammation of both tympanic membranes (Fig. 3-2) and congestion of the nasopharynx is noted.

This is the classic presentation of otitis media. As noted above, the predisposition to otitis media is based on anatomic considerations. In addition, the increased incidence of upper respiratory infections in the pediatric age group is also responsible for the noted increased incidence of ear infections. The treatment of acute otitis media has changed over the years. Bacterial infection involving *Hemophilus influenza* and *Streptococcal pneumoniae* are common causes of otitis media; however, it is recognized that a substantial number are caused by viral infection. In the past, antibiotic therapy was the mainstay of treatment; however, more recently, studies have questioned the use of antibiotics in the initial management of simple cases of otitis media. Initial treatment with analgesics such as ibuprofen and decongestants is often recommended initially in children over six months who are in otherwise good health. If no improvement is noted, then antibiotics are instituted. In reality, most clinicians treat almost all cases of otitis media with antibiotics in clinical practice. There are two main reasons: First and most important, the parents often want immediate treatment of their child, and second, most parents would find it difficult to return if symptoms don't improve, since that would require them to take time off from work or other responsibilities to see the doctor.

When to recommend surgery for otitis media remains controversial. Repeated episodes of otitis media may produce temporary hearing problems that, with time, can become permanent due to scarring. To prevent hearing loss at a very crucial time in the infant's learning process is the primary aim. One of the common causes of school problems and learning in the pediatric patient are problems associated with hearing, often due to chronic otitis media. The usual surgical procedure performed, when medical treatment fails, is adenoidectomy and tube placement (Fig. 3-3). The adenoids are lymphatic tissue located close to the Eustachian tube. When infection occurs, especially in the upper respiratory tract, these tissues swell, obstructing the tube and limiting drainage from the middle ear, thus allowing overgrowth of bacteria. By placing a tube in the middle ear, the fluid and infection can drain freely into the external auditory canal, preventing otitis media. If recurrent streptococcal pharyngitis is present, tonsillectomy may be recommended.

Figure 3-3. Foreign body in the upper airway. (From Osborn LM, DeWitt TG, First LR, Zenel JA: *Pediatrics*. St. Louis, Mosby, 2005.)

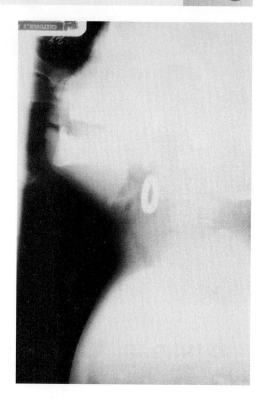

FOLLOW-UP

English	Spanish Formal	Spanish Informal
Ms. Rivas, based on the history and physical exam, I believe Denise has an ear infection. This can cause fever as can the upper respiratory infection that she has. I am going to recommend antibiotics because of her young age. It should take about 24 hours for the fever to start coming down. She should be given Tylenol alternating with ibuprofen to ease the pain and bring down the fever. It is important to call us if there is any worsening of the fever after 24 hours.	Sra. Rivas, de acuerdo con la historia y los resultados del examen físico, yo pienso que Denise tiene una infección de oído. Esta infección le puede causar fiebre, al igual que la infección respiratoria que ella tiene. Como está pequeña *(chiquita)*, le voy a recomendar antibióticos. La fiebre debe comenzar a bajar dentro de unas veinticuatro horas. Hay que darle Tylenol e Ibuprofen alternativamente para aliviar el dolor y bajar la fiebre. Es importante que nos llame si la fiebre aumenta después de veinticuatro horas.	Sra. Rivas, creo que Denise tiene una infección de oído. La infección de oído y la gripe le pueden causar la calentura. Le voy a mandar un antibiótico para la infección. La calentura le debe bajar de hoy a mañana. También hay que darle Tylenol e Ibuprofén para quitarle el dolor y bajar la calentura. Quiero que me llame mañana en la tarde si la calentura sigue subiendo.
Also, if she stops taking in fluids, we need to be called. Most likely you will see an improvement in 24 hours. We need to see you both back in 10 days to examine Denise's ears for follow-up, even though she should be better by then.	También tiene que llamarnos si Denise deja de tomar líquidos. Lo más probable es que ella mejorará en las próximas veinticuatro horas. Quiero verlas de nuevo en diez días para examinar los oídos de Denise, aunque ella debería estar bien para entonces.	También quiero que me llame si Denise deja de tomar aguas frescas. Pero yo creo que va a mejorar de hoy para mañana. De todas maneras, quiero ver a Denise en diez días para examinarle los oídos una vez más.

The key to treating an emergency is not always that we diagnose and treat the illness perfectly the first time—we are human and make mistakes—but follow-up is crucial. That we explain to our patient's mother what to expect, to call if there is no improvement or if the condition worsens, is important. Follow-up is also critical in this patient due to the fact that hearing loss may be present if our patient develops repeated episodes of ear infections. Surgical referral may be necessary at a later date.

CASE 2: EPIGLOTTITIS

CHIEF COMPLAINT

A 5-year-old boy presents with a chief complaint of fever, cough, and respiratory distress.

As you enter the room, you notice the patient is breathing rapidly and with great effort. He is sitting up in bed and there is saliva (secretions) coming out of the child's mouth. (You introduce yourself quickly.) There is nasal flaring and the patient is using the accessory muscles of respiration (the sternocleido-mastoid muscles). You can hear inspiratory stridor during respirations. (Stridor is a sound produced during breathing due to air moving through a narrowed tube. When severe, it is often audible without a stethoscope. It is harsh and high-pitched, very different from the soft, normal breath sounds of unlabored breathing.) There is cyanosis noted around the lips. What is your next step?

Fortunately, even in an emergency room, most situations encountered are not emergent, i.e., there is time to do a focused history and physical exam prior to coming to a diagnosis. That is not the case here. In trauma surgery, we always teach the ABCs of trauma: Airway, Breathing, Circulation. These are addressed before anything, including history and physical exam (what good does it do if your patient is not breathing and you're trying to do a history?). In our patient there is severe respiratory distress, as manifested by cyanosis, nasal flaring, and the use of accessory respiratory muscles. This has to be addressed immediately. In other words, this is a life-threatening situation. A rapid respiratory rate in the pediatric population is a common finding. Children can increase their respiratory rates to incredible levels compared to adults due to their incredible ability to maintain this increased "work" effort; this is a common finding in children with respiratory infections and conditions such as asthma.

However, in this case, of great concern is the stridor, the nasal flaring, the use of accessory muscles of respiration, and cyanosis. When the child inspires, the nasal cartilages widen, reflecting an increased effort to inspire a greater volume of oxygen. The accessory muscle of respiration, i.e., the neck muscle, attaches to the sternum and first rib and helps expand the rib cage, promoting inspiration. Again, this is not a normal finding and indicates severe problems with respiration and hypoxemia. Cyanosis is of grave concern, indicating hypoxemia—the bluish tinge of the patient's skin is due to hemoglobin unbound by oxygen. It is best seen around the lips and under the fingernails. Finally, stridor can be seen in a number of upper respiratory infectious conditions and is always of concern due to the fact that it indicates some narrowing of the upper respiratory tract, i.e., the larynx and/or trachea. Coupled with the physical findings above, this represents a true airway emergency. There is urgency in treating this life-threatening problem.

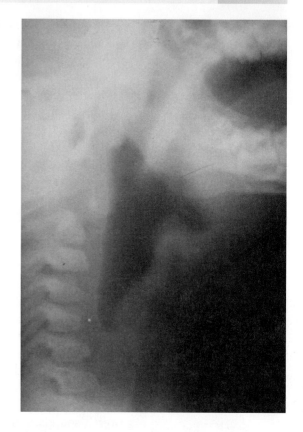

Figure 3-4. Lateral neck radiograph in a child with epiglottitis. (From Long S, Pickering L, Prober C: *Principles and Practice of Pediatric Infectious Diseases*, ed 2. Philadelphia, Churchill Livingstone, 2003.)

The challenge is to make the diagnosis as quickly as possible and initiate therapy. Thus, questions are initially focused on making the diagnosis urgently. Respiratory distress in the pediatric patient is most often caused by: (1) Upper-airway obstruction, involving the supra- and infra-glottic region due to a foreign body such as a swallowed coin or peanut, epiglottitis (an infection and inflammation of the glottic region; Fig. 3-4), and infections of the trachea and proximal bronchii by viruses termed croup; (2) Lower airway disease affecting the distal bronchus and lungs. These conditions such as pneumonia, asthma, and bronchitis are very common in the pediatric patient. However, stridor is a classic finding in upper airway obstruction.

HISTORY AND PHYSICAL EXAM

	English	Spanish Formal	Spanish Informal
	Hi, Ms. Thomas, I am Robert Smith, a fourth year medical student working with Dr. Jones. Your child is having difficulty breathing so I want to examine him before we go into a detailed history.	Hola, Srta. Thomas, soy Robert Smith, estudiante de medicina de cuarto año. Trabajo con el Dr. Jones. Como su hijo tiene dificultad para respirar, lo voy a examinar antes de hacerle una historia detallada.	Hola, Srta. Thomas, me llamo Robert Smith. Soy estudiante de medicina de cuarto año que trabaja con el Dr. Jones. Como su hijo no puede respirar bien, lo voy a examinar antes de hacerle la historia clínica.
Q.	Does he have asthma or any other lung problems? Is there any chance he may have swallowed anything?	¿Padece de asma o algún otro problema de los pulmones? ¿Hay alguna posibilidad de que se haya tragado algo?	¿Tiene algún problema de los pulmones, como asma? ¿Cree que tal vez se tragó algo?
A.	He has frequent colds but doesn't have asthma and I don't think he has swallowed anything.	Él se resfría con frecuencia, pero no padece de asma y no creo que se haya tragado nada.	Tiene catarro con frecuencia pero nunca ha tenido asma. No creo que se haya tragado nada.

	English	Spanish Formal	Spanish Informal
Q.	(To the five-year-old child): What is your name?	(Al niño de cinco años): ¿Cuál es tu nombre?	¿Cómo te llamas?
A.	Robert. (The response is clear.)	Roberto. (La respuesta es clara.)	Roberto.
Q.	Robert, I am going to listen to your heart and lungs real fast with this (points to the stethoscope.) This won't hurt at all. Is that ok?	Roberto, te voy a escuchar el corazón y los pulmones rapidito (*rápidamente*) con esto (señala el estetoscopio), no te va a doler nada. ¿Está bien?	Roberto, voy a oírte el corazón y los pulmones con esto (señala el estetoscopio), no va a doler nada. ¿De acuerdo?
A.	OK.	Está bien.	De acuerdo.

You note good breath sounds bilaterally. There are no wheezes, crackles, or rhonchi. However, pronounced stridor is noted. This is a very serious situation. Based on this rapid exam performed in less than 60 seconds, you have ruled out a lower airway problem such as pneumonia or asthma. No wheezes are noted, making asthma unlikely, and no rales or rhonchi are noted, making pneumonia and bronchitis unlikely. The observation of stridor, a sound made by obstruction of the upper airway, is most likely. The fact that the child can speak clearly makes laryngitis less likely, for in this disease the patient often loses his or her voice. Of great concern is epiglottitis due to the upper-airway obstruction and the fever. This is also the most common age for the disease. You don't want to look into the child's pharynx because this may initiate laryngospasm. Lateral x-rays can confirm the diagnosis (see Fig. 3-4). This is most often caused by *Hemophilus influenza*. An ear, nose, and throat (ENT) consult is obtained emergently as is anesthesiology to establish an airway if the child is in severe distress, as in this case. Intubation can be extremely difficult due to obstruction by the swollen epiglottis.

FOLLOW-UP

English	Spanish Formal	Spanish Informal
Ms. Thomas, I believe Robert has an infection of the opening of where the air enters the tube leading to the lung. This is called epiglottitis. It can be treated by antibiotics, but because of the severe problems breathing, we are calling two specialists to come and see Robert.	Srta. Thomas, yo pienso que Roberto tiene una infección del orificio por donde entra el aire al tubo que va para los pulmones. Se llama epiglotitis. Se puede tratar con antibióticos, pero por la gran dificultad que tiene para respirar, vamos a llamar a dos especialistas para que vengan a verlo.	Srta. Thomas, creo que Roberto tiene una infección del tubo que va para los pulmones, se llama epiglotitis. Se puede tratar con antibióticos, pero como le cuesta tanto respirar, vamos a llamar a dos especialistas para que lo vean.
Temporarily, he may need to have a tube put in his throat to help him breathe until the infection and swelling goes down, which usually takes two or three days. The specialist will make that decision based on how much inflammation is present in the upper part of the airway or lungs.	Temporalmente, va a necesitar que le pongamos un tubo en la garganta para ayudarle a respirar hasta que la infección y la inflamación disminuyan. Por lo general, esto toma dos o tres días. El especialista tomará la decisión en base a la cantidad de inflamación presente en las vías aéreas o los pulmones.	Por ahora, va a necesitar un tubo en la garganta para ayudarle a respirar hasta que la infección y la inflamación disminuyan. Esto dura por lo general dos o tres días. El especialista decidirá de acuerdo a la inflamación que tenga en las vías aéreas o los pulmones.

In the pediatric patient, the decision to intubate your patient is most often made on clinical grounds, i.e., the degree of respiratory distress, as seen in this case by the use of accessory muscles of respiration, severe stridor, and cyanosis. Blood gas analysis in the child is much less helpful than in the adult. Following admission to the hospital and treatment with antibiotics, complete recovery is expected. The child is usually intubated and placed on a ventilator if severe obstruction is present for about 48 hours.

CASE 3: GASTROENTERITIS

CHIEF COMPLAINT

A six-month-old girl presents with fever, vomiting, and diarrhea of three days duration.

HISTORY

English	Spanish Formal	Spanish Informal
Hello, Mr. Lopez, my name is Isabel Rapa, I am a third year medical student working with Dr. Mohr. I will ask you some questions and then do a brief exam, and Dr. Mohr will be in following this.	Hola, Sr. López, mi nombre es Isabel Rapa. Soy estudiante de medicina de tercer año que trabaja con el Dr. Mohr. Le voy a hacer algunas preguntas y después un examen breve. El Dr. Mohr vendrá después.	Hola, Sr. López, me llamo Isabel Rapa. Soy estudiante de medicina de tercer año. Trabajo con el Dr. Mohr. Le voy a hacer unas preguntas y después la voy a examinar. El Dr. Mohr vendrá después.
Q. What brings you in to see us today?	¿Por qué viene a vernos hoy?	¿Por qué vino hoy?
A. My daughter Annabelle has been vomiting for the past three days. She can't eat anything without vomiting.	Mi hija Annabelle ha estado vomitando los últimos tres días. No puede comer nada porque lo vomita.	Annabelle, mi hija, tiene tres días de estar vomitando. No para nada en el estómago.
Q. Has she had diarrhea?	¿Ha tenido diarrea?	¿Ha estado floja del estómago?
A. Yes, this started about two days ago.	Sí, le comenzó hace como dos días.	Sí, empezó hace un par de días.
Q. Has she had fever and if so, how high?	¿Ha tenido fiebre? Y de ser así, ¿qué tan alta?	¿Ha tenido fiebre? ¿Cuánto le ha subido?
A. She has had fever to 102 degrees and we have been giving her Tylenol.	Ha tenido ciento dos grados de temperatura y le hemos estado dando Tylenol.	Tenía ciento dos grados. Le hemos estado dando Tylenol.
Q. Does she breast feed?	¿Le está dando leche de pecho?	¿Le está dando de mamar?
A. No, she takes formula and regular food.	No, está tomando leche de fórmula (en polvo) y comida regular.	No, está tomando leche de tarro y comida regular.
Q. Is she taking liquids? And what kind of liquids are you giving her?	¿Está tomando líquidos? ¿Y qué tipo de líquidos le están dando?	¿Está tomando líquidos? ¿Y qué le están dando?
A. She holds some liquids down. We are giving her formula and fruit juices.	Está sosteniendo una poco de líquidos. Le estamos dando fórmula y jugos de fruta.	Está sosteniendo líquidos un poco. Ha estado tomando leche de tarro y jugos de fruta.
Q. Is she peeing as much as before?	¿Está orinando igual que antes?	¿Orina igual que antes?
A. No, we change the diaper because of the diarrhea.	No, le cambiamos el pañal por la diarrea.	No, la cambiamos por la diarrea.
Q. Have you noticed tears when she cries?	¿Ha notado lágrimas cuando llora?	¿Tiene lágrimas cuando llora?

	English	Spanish Formal	Spanish Informal
A.	Yes, but not as much as before.	Sí, pero no tanto como antes.	Sí, pero menos que antes.
Q.	Have you noted any blood or mucous in the diarrhea?	¿Ha notado sangre o moco en la diarrea?	¿Ha tenido moco o sangre en los excrementos?
A.	No, I haven't seen any mucous or blood in the diarrhea.	No, no he visto sangre ni moco en la diarrea.	No.
Q.	Is anyone sick at home?	¿Hay alguien enfermo en su casa?	¿Hay algún enfermo en la casa?
A.	No, no one is sick at home.	No, nadie está enfermo en la casa.	No.
Q.	Have you traveled anywhere recently?	¿Han viajado a algún lugar recientemente?	¿Y ha viajado recientemente?
A.	We traveled to Mexico about two weeks ago. We stayed about three days.	Viajamos a México hace como dos semanas. Nos quedamos como tres días.	Fuimos a México hace dos semanas. Estuvimos allá como tres días.
Q.	Has she had a history of recurrent attacks of diarrhea or vomiting?	¿Ha padecido de ataques de diarrea o vómito frecuentemente en el pasado?	¿Ha tenido ataques de diarrea o vómito frecuente en el pasado?
A.	No, she has not had problems with diarrhea in the past.	No, no ha tenido problemas de diarrea anteriormente.	No.
Q.	Has she been active or has she been sleeping most of the time?	¿Ha estado activa o ha estado durmiendo la mayor parte del tiempo?	¿Está activa o muy dormilona?
A.	She is active but when she gets the fever she gets real sleepy.	Está activa, pero cuando le da fiebre, le da mucho sueño.	Está juguetona, pero cuando le sube la calentura, le da sólo por dormir.
Q.	Does she act hungry and want to eat?	¿Parece que tuviera hambre y quiere comer?	¿Parece que tuviera ganas de comer?
A.	Yes, she cries for the bottle but we are afraid to give her too much because of the vomiting.	Sí, llora por el biberón (la botella), pero nos da miedo darle demasiado por los vómitos.	Sí, llora por la botella (pacha, chupón), pero no queremos darle mucho por los vómitos.
Q.	Does she have abdominal pain? Does she hold her stomach and cry for periods of time?	¿Tiene dolor de panza (abdomen)? ¿Se sostiene el estómago y llora por un rato (periodos de tiempo)?	¿Le duele el estómago? ¿Se sostiene la panza y llora de vez en cuando?
A.	She cries when she has gone to the bathroom, more than anything when the diaper needs changing. She doesn't have fits of crying and holding her stomach.	Llora cuando ha dado del cuerpo, pero más que nada cuando hay que cambiarle el pañal. No tiene ataques en que llora y se sostiene el estómago.	Llora cuando ha hecho "pu, pu", pero más cuando hay que cambiarla. No tiene ataques en que llora y se sostiene el estómago.
Q.	Is she getting better?	¿Está mejorando?	¿Parece mejor?
A.	She is about the same.	Está casi igual que antes.	Parecido a antes.
	Mr. Lopez, I am going to do a physical exam. Can you hold the baby and I will examine the heart, lungs, and stomach first and then the throat and ears?	Sr. Lopez, voy a hacer un examen físico. ¿Puede sostener a la niña para examinarle el corazón, los pulmones y el estómago primero, y después los oídos y la garganta?	Sr. Lopez, voy a hacerle un examen físico. ¿Puede sostener a Annabelle para examinarle el corazón, los pulmones y el estómago primero, y después los oídos y la garganta?

THE PHYSICAL EXAM

Physical exam reveals very dry mucous membranes and minimal tear formation as the baby cries. The rest of the exam is normal. The baby is active and readily drinks an electrolyte solution bottle you give her and holds it down without vomiting.

DIFFERENTIAL DIAGNOSIS

This is one of the most common causes of a visit to the Emergency Room or urgent care setting—diarrhea and vomiting. The most common cause of this is viral gastroenteritis. Often vomiting is present first and progresses to involve the lower part of the gastrointestinal tract. Often fever is present. Recent travel may increase the suspicion for a bacterial cause of the gastroenteritis such as infections with *Shigella*, *salmonella*, and *E. coli*. Although not 100% correct, patients with gastroenteritis due to bacterial infection versus viral may present with blood and mucous (pus) in the stool, often visible when the diaper is changed.

Although a much rarer cause of the above clinical presentation, appendicitis always has to be in your differential diagnosis. In appendicitis, the child will have a very poor appetite and is often distended on physical exam of the abdomen, due to an ileus or a non-mechanical obstruction caused by inhibition of peristalsis by the inflamed, often perforated appendix. In this age group, appendicitis often presents late with perforation due to the inability of the child to communicate his or her symptoms.

The above clinical presentation is very consistent with viral gastroenteritis. Of note are the dry mucous membranes and minimal tear formation suggestive of dehydration. Occasionally, infants of this age need to be admitted for intravenous hydration if the diarrhea and vomiting is severe. This is often a tough call and is based on a number of factors. Age is a crucial one. Babies under six months of age are much more likely to get into trouble with severe dehydration than older pediatric patients. This is due to a number of factors, including the inability to concentrate the urine well and the loss of free water in the younger infant. Also, the intravascular volume in the infant is much lower than in the child over a year of age, predisposing them to more severe degrees of hypovolemia with comparable volume loss. Infants over the age of one year have much more reserve than younger infants, allowing us as clinicians to try a trial of treatment on an outpatient basis. This case is a tough call because the baby has obvious evidence of dehydration. However, she is producing tears and is an older infant. Often we will give babies clear liquids in the emergency room to observe their ability to take fluids as well as to observe the response afterward. In this case, the baby has held down the electrolyte solution. With reliable parents, she can be monitored at home. It is important to instruct the parents not to give any solid foods for the first 48 hours and no milk products for the first few days. Lactase is lost due to the inflammation of the intestinal mucosa, so lactose is poorly absorbed. Usually, we recommend clear liquids such as Gatorade, jello, chicken broth, etc., i.e., things that allow the light to shine through. This allows the intestinal villi to regenerate.

FOLLOW-UP

English	Spanish Formal	Spanish Informal
I believe Annabelle has gastroenteritis, an inflammation of the lining of the intestine. It is important to give her only clear liquids for the first few days. As the vomiting and diarrhea improve by the third day you can introduce bland solid foods	Yo pienso que Annabelle tiene gastroenteritis, una inflamación del revestimiento de los intestinos. Es importante darle solamente líquidos claros los primeros días. Conforme mejoren los vómitos y la diarrea, para el tercer día, puede comenzar a darle	Creo que Annabelle tiene gastroenteritis, una inflamación de los intestinos. Es importante darle sólo líquidos claros los primeros días. Para el tercer día, cuando mejoren los vómitos y la diarrea, puede empezar a darle comidas suaves,

English	Spanish Formal	Spanish Informal
such as white rice, boiled potatoes, etc. I would wait at least three days before introducing milk products. We would like you to call in 24 hours to let us know how Annabelle is doing. If she cannot hold any of the liquids down or things get worse call us sooner. Are there any questions that you have?	comidas blandas, como arroz blanco, papas hervidas, etc. Yo esperaría por lo menos tres días antes de comenzar a darle leche (productos lácteos). Quiero que nos llame en veinticuatro horas para decirnos cómo está Annabelle. Si no puede sostener los líquidos o se pone peor, llámenos antes. ¿Tiene alguna pregunta?	como arroz blanco y papas hervidas. Yo esperaría al menos tres días antes de darle leche. Llámenos en veinticuatro horas para saber cómo está Annabelle. Si se pone peor, llámenos antes. ¿Tiene preguntas?
Q. Are you sure that it is not something more serious?	¿Está segura de que no es algo más serio?	No, pero ¿está segura de que no es más grave?
A. We can never be 100% sure but the symptoms that Annabelle has and the physical exam make this most likely. That is why we want to hear from you in 24 hours. If things are not getting better we want to see her back.	Nunca podemos estar ciento por ciento seguros, pero por los síntomas que tiene Annabelle y los resultados del examen físico, es lo más probable. Por eso queremos que nos llame en veinticuatro horas. Si las cosas no están mejorando, vamos a querer verla otra vez.	Nunca podemos estar completamente seguros, pero por los síntomas y los resultados del examen, es lo más probable. Por eso queremos que nos llame en veinticuatro horas. Si las cosas no mejoran, vamos a tener que verla otra vez.

The key in situations such as the above case is to have an open avenue of communication. In other words, follow-up. If by 24 hours there is no improvement, you may want to re-evaluate this patient. At times admission is necessary to infuse intravenous fluids, allowing the infection to pass and the intestinal villi to regenerate. In addition, say the patient has appendicitis (an unlikely event based on the history and physical exam). By telling the parent to call if there is a worsening of the child's condition, you have encouraged open communication. We cannot be right in our diagnosis all the time. The other important key is that if you have concerns about the follow-up, then sometimes it is safer to admit the patient.

CASE 4: LACERATION

CHIEF COMPLAINT

A seven-year-old boy presents to the emergency room with a laceration of the hand. Because lacerations are common in children, especially at this age, the questioning is a bit different in terms of the focused history and physical exam.

HISTORY

English	Spanish Formal	Spanish Informal
Q. Hello, Mr. Jefferson, hello Tom, I am Dr. Belsher. (To Tom): What happened to you, Tom?	Hola, Sr. Jefferson. Hola Tom, soy el Dra. Belsher. (A Tom): ¿Qué sucedió, Tom?	Hola, Sr. Jefferson. Hola Tom, soy la Dra. Belsher. (A Tom): ¿Qué pasó, Tom?
A. I was trying to cut an apple and the knife slipped.	Estaba tratando de partir una manzana y se me resbaló el cuchillo.	Estaba partiendo una manzana y se me escurrió el cuchillo.
Q. How long ago did it happen?	¿Hace cuánto sucedió?	¿Cuándo pasó?
A. About two hours ago.	Hace como dos horas.	Hace dos horas.

	English	Spanish Formal	Spanish Informal Continued
Q.	What did you do then?	¿Qué hiciste después?	¿Y luego qué hiciste?
A.	My dad wrapped it in a towel and we came to the emergency room.	Mi papá me envolvió la herida con una toalla y nos vinimos para el servicio de emergencias.	Mi papá me cubrió con un paño y nos vinimos para emergencias.
Q.	Did it bleed a lot?	¿Tuviste mucho sangrado?	¿Sangraste mucho?
A.	At first it bled a lot, but after it was wrapped, it stopped, I think.	Al principio sangró mucho, pero después de envolverlo, dejó de sangrar.	Me salió mucha sangre al principio, pero después de cubrirlo, dejó de sangrar.
Q.	Do you feel light headed or funny when you stand?	¿Sientes ganas de desmayarte o raro cuando estás de pie?	¿Te sientes raro o como que te vas a desmayar?
A.	At first, I thought I would faint when I saw the blood but I feel better now.	Al principio pensé que me iba a desmayar cuando vi la sangre, pero ahora me siento mejor.	Ahora estoy mejor, pero al principio pensé que me iba a desmayar cuando vi la sangre.
Q.	Was it spurting or bleeding real heavy?	¿Estaba sangrando mucho?	¿Te salía como un chorro?
A.	At first it was bleeding real hard but then my mom put pressure on it and it slowed down. Father: The blood was spurting out and then I put pressure on it and it slowed down.	Al principio estaba sangrando mucho, pero después, cuando papá aplicó presión, empezó a sangrar menos. Papá: Estaba sangrando mucho, pero después le apliqué presión y se redujo.	Primero era como un chorro, pero después, cuando papá le puso presión, era menos. Papá: La sangre salía a chorros, pero después le puse presión y disminuyó.
Q.	How are you feeling now?	¿Cómo te sientes ahora?	¿Cómo te sientes?
A.	I am scared about getting stitches. Is it going to hurt?	Tengo miedo de que me cosan. ¿Me va a doler?	Me da miedo que me cosan. ¿Me va a doler?
A.	(To Tom): We will make the cut numb with some medicine so if we need to put stitches in it won't hurt.	(A Tom): Vamos a dormir la herida con una medicina así que no te va a doler si tenemos que ponerle la costura.	(A Tom): Te vamos a poner una medicina para dormirte la cortada. Así que no va a doler si tenemos que coserte.
Q.	(To the father): Are Tom's immunizations up to date? Do you know when he had his last tetanus shot?	(Al padre): ¿Tom tiene todas las vacunas al día? ¿Se acuerda cuándo le pusieron la última vacuna para el tétano?	(Al padre): ¿Tom está al día con las vacunas? ¿Cuándo le pusieron la última vacuna para el tétano?
A.	I'm not sure. I know he had a tetanus shot this year before starting school.	No estoy seguro si le pusieron la vacuna del tétano este año antes de comenzar la escuela.	No estoy seguro si lo vacunaron contra el tétano este año antes de empezar la escuela.
Q.	Tom, do the hand and finger tips feel funny like they are asleep?	Tom, ¿la mano y la punta de los dedos se sienten raros, como si estuvieran dormidos?	¿Tom, sientes como si tuvieras dormidos la mano y las puntas de los dedos?
A.	No, it feels normal.	No, los siento normal.	No.
Q.	Can you move your fingers normally?	¿Puedes mover los dedos normalmente?	¿Puedes mover los dedos?
A.	Yes, I can move my fingers but it hurts where I got cut.	Sí, puedo mover los dedos, pero me duele donde tengo la cortada.	Sí, pero me duele la cortada.
Q.	(To Tom's father): Does Tom have any medical problems such as heart or lung disease?	(Al papá de Tom): ¿Tom padece de algún problema de salud, como del corazón o de los pulmones?	(Al papá de Tom): ¿Tom tiene algún otro problema, como del corazón o de los pulmones?
A.	No, not now. He did have bronchitis when he was four years old and they hospitalized him.	No, ahora no. Tuvo bronquitis cuando tenía cuatro años y lo internaron en el hospital.	No. Estuvo en el hospital cuando tenía cuatro años por una bronquitis.
Q.	Does he take any medicines?	¿Toma alguna medicina?	¿Está tomando alguna medicina?
A.	No, he doesn't take any medications except for an occasional ibuprofen when he gets a headache.	No, no toma ninguna medicina, excepto por Ibuprofen de vez en cuando, cuando tiene dolor de cabeza.	No, solo Ibuprofen de vez en cuando, cuando le duele la cabeza.

	English	Spanish Formal	Spanish Informal
Q.	Does he have any allergies?	¿Tiene algún tipo de alergia?	¿Padece de alergias?
A.	Yes, he got penicillin once and had a rash.	Sí, una vez tuvo un brote cuando le dieron penicilina.	Sí, se brotó en un salpullido una vez cuando le dieron penicilina.

In the physical exam, we will focus on the laceration. We want to know if there is any bone, tendon, nerve, or arterial injury. If this is the case, we have to call in a specialist such as an orthopedic or plastic surgeon with a specialty in hand injuries. In this case, the cut is on the palmer or volar surface of the hand. Location helps us determine the possible injuries that might have occurred. Lacerations on the ventral or volar surface of the hand and forearm are much more worrisome than dorsal lacerations. On the volar aspect of the forearm and hand, we have the flexor tendons, the median and ulnar nerves, and the radial and ulnar arteries Fig. 3-5. On the dorsal surface, we have the extensor tendons and the radial

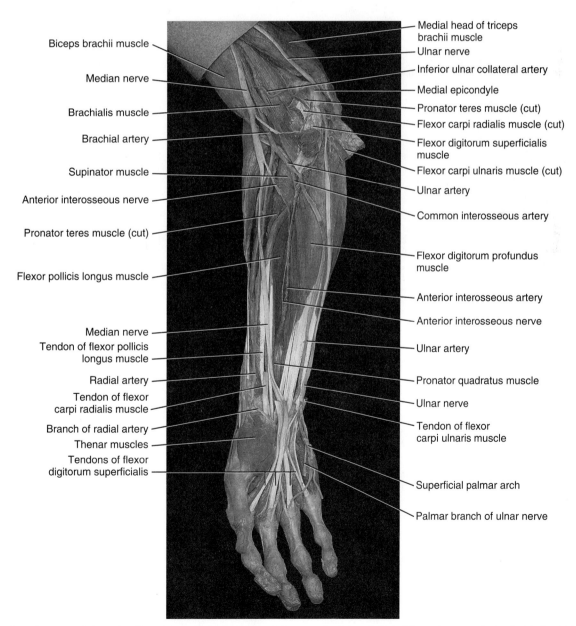

Figure 3-5. Anatomy of the wrist. (From Moses K, Banks J, Nava P, Petersen D: *Atlas of Clinical Gross Anatomy.* St. Louis, Mosby, 2005.)

nerves, which are sensory nerves at the level of the wrist. The median nerve and ulnar nerve are crucial motor and sensory nerves to the hand and forearm, and injury to these can result in major disability. In addition, flexor tendons function in fine motor movement of the fingers, while the extensor tendons function in extending the fingers and are much less involved with fine motor movements. Thus, our exam will involve testing sensory and motor functions of the median and ulnar nerves, testing flexor tendon function, and assessing pulses.

PHYSICAL EXAM

	English	Spanish Formal	Spanish Informal
	Tom, I am going to examine the cut, I will be real gentle. I need to unwrap the dressing.	Tom, voy a examinar la cortada. Lo voy a hacer con mucho cuidado, tengo que quitar el vendaje.	Tom, tengo que examinarte la herida. Lo voy a hacer con cuidado, tengo que quitarte la venda.
	(A 3-centimeter cut is noted at the wrist on the volar aspect. It is not bleeding at present).		
Q.	Tom, I am going to examine your hand to see if anything deep has been cut, OK?	Tom, voy a examinar la mano para ver si se cortó alguna otra cosa profundamente. ¿Está bien?	Tengo que examinar la mano para ver si se cortó algo en la parte de adentro. ¿Está bien?
Q.	Will it hurt?	¿Me va a doler?	¿Me va a doler?
A.	No, I am just going to ask you to move your fingers and touch your skin to see if any nerve has been injured.	No, sólo te voy a pedir que muevas los dedos y te voy a tocar la piel para ver si hay algún nervio afectado.	No, sólo te voy a decir que muevas los dedos y los voy a tocar para ver si hay algún nervio dañado.
Q.	(Touching the volar surface of the fingers, alternating the injured side with the normal side.) Can you feel this, Tom, and does it feel the same as the other side? (You are testing median nerve and ulnar nerve sensory function.)	¿Puedes sentir esto, Tom? ¿Se siente igual que en el otro lado?	¿Sientes esto, Tom? ¿Sientes igual que en el otro lado?
A.	Yes, I can feel you touching me and it feels the same.	Sí, puedo sentir cuando me toca y se siente igual.	Sí, siento cuando me toca y se siente igual.
Q.	I am going to have you bend and straighten each finger by itself. Bend and straighten your thumb (next index, middle, ring, and little finger; that is what they are called in medical terminology).	Te voy a pedir que dobles y endereces cada dedo a la vez. Dobla y endereza el dedo pulgar (después el índice, medio, anular, y meñique).	Voy a pedirte que dobles y endereces cada dedo a la vez. Dobla y endereza el dedo gordo (después el índice, corazón, anular y meñique).
	(Here we are testing flexor tendon function—the ability to flex the fingers at metacarpal-phalangeal joint and the proximal and distal interphalangeal joints.)		
	Next, I am going to check your pulses to make sure the blood vessels are OK.	Ahora te voy a palpar los pulsos para estar seguro de que los vasos sanguíneos están bien.	Ahora voy a tocar los pulsos para asegurarme de que los vasos sanguíneos estén bien.

English	Spanish Formal	Spanish Informal
(Here we palpate the radial and ulnar arterial pulse, always comparing both sides. A difference in magnitude of one side compared to the other often indicates an arterial injury. Due to collateral circulation with arterial injury, one might feel a pulse on the injured side but it is usually diminished in amplitude.)		
Both pulses are strong.	Ambos pulsos son fuertes.	Los dos se sienten fuertes.
(To the Dad and to Tom): I have good news. There is no evidence of nerve, tendon, or arterial injury. I am going to numb up the cut with an anesthetic, Xylocaine.	(Al papá y a Tom): Tengo buenas noticias. No hay evidencia de lesión del nervio, el tendón o la arteria. Le voy a dormir la herida con un anestésico, xilocaína.	(Al papá y a Tom): Tengo buenas noticias. No hay evidencia de que el nervio, el tendón o la arteria estén dañados. Le voy a dormir la cortada con un anestésico que se llama xilocaína.
Tom, I am going to give you a shot that will make the cut go numb so when we sew the cut up you won't feel any pain. The shot will sting for a few seconds then you won't feel anything.	Tom, te voy a poner una inyección que va a dormir la herida para que cuando la cosamos no sientas dolor. La inyección te va a escocer por unos segundos, pero después no vas a sentir nada.	Tom, te voy a poner una inyección para dormirte la cortada y para que no sientas cuando la estemos cosiendo. La inyección va a picar un poco, pero después no vas a sentir nada.
(Injecting the local anesthetic)		
Tom, hold real still while I do the injection. Then it will be numb and you won't feel anything when we sew the cut closed.	Tom, estate quieto mientras te inyecto. Después la herida se va a dormir y no sentirás nada cuando te cosamos.	No te muevas mientras te inyecto. Después se te va a dormir la herida y no vas a sentir nada cuando la cosemos.

The follow-up after closing the wound is very important. Of primary importance is the risk of wound infection. After sewing closed any laceration, there is a 5% to 10% risk of wound infection.

It is lower in well-vascularized areas such as the head and neck region, and highest in regions of diminished perfusion such as the distal extremities (i.e., hands and feet). This is especially true in older patients who have a long history of smoking with concomitant atherosclerosis. It is also related to the time between when the accident occurred and when you are closing the wound. In general, wounds greater than 6 to 12 hours old are often left open to heal by what we call secondary intention. After 6 hours, the inoculum of bacteria starts to increase and closing the wound increases the risk of wound infection. In other words, the wound is cleaned and the patient is instructed to clean the wound twice a day and pack it with moist gauze pads. Slowly, granulation tissue is laid down and wound contraction occurs, closing the wound. By allowing the wound to heal by this manner, wound infection is much less likely than if you close the wound, termed primary intention. Finally, the mechanism of injury is important. Wounds caused by human and dog bites carry a high risk of infection if the wound is closed. Other than face lacerations, these kinds of wounds are generally left open. We caution patients as to the symptoms of wound infection and to return if this is suspected. These generally present at about 5 days with redness around the wound, increasing pain, and fever. If any of these occur, we encourage the patient to seek medical advice.

FOLLOW-UP

English	Spanish Formal	Spanish Informal
Everything looks good. The wound is closed. You may take the dressing off in 24 hours and you can clean the wound with soap and water.	Todo se ve bien. La herida está cerrada. Se puede quitar el vendaje en veinticuatro horas y puede lavarse la herida con agua y jabón.	Todo se ve bien. La cortada está cerrada. Se puede quitar la venda dentro de veinticuatro horas y puede lavarse con agua y jabón.
Q. (Dad): Does he have to have a dressing over the wound after he cleans it?	(Papá): ¿Tiene que ponerse una venda sobre la herida después de limpiarla?	(Papá): ¿Tiene que volverse a vendar después de limpiar la herida?
A. No, the wound is sealed by 24 hours, but for safety so he doesn't bump it and cosmetically it is sometimes more comfortable to have it covered.	No, la herida va a estar cerrada en veinticuatro horas, pero para más seguridad, para que no se la golpee, y porque desde el punto de vista cosmético, a veces es más cómodo tenerla cubierta.	No, la herida va a estar cerrada en veinticuatro horas, pero para estar seguros de que no se va a golpear, a veces es más cómodo tenerla cubierta.
We will have you back in a week to remove the stitches. It is important that if the wound becomes red or if there is increasing pain around the wound or fever to call our office and we will see you sooner.	Vamos a verlo otra vez en una semana para quitar las costuras. Es importante que si la herida se pone de color rojo o si tiene mucho dolor o fiebre, llame a la oficina para verlo otra vez.	Lo queremos ver en una semana para quitarle las costuras. Si la cortada se pone roja o si siente mucho dolor o calentura, tiene que llamarnos y venir otra vez lo más pronto posible.
These might be signs of a wound infection and we would want to see you sooner. The risk of this is about 1 in 10 to 1 in 20.	Estos pueden ser signos de infección de la herida y lo vamos a querer ver otra vez. El riesgo de infección es de uno en diez a uno en veinte.	Puede ser que tenga una infección y, en ese caso, lo tenemos que ver otra vez. El riesgo de infección es de una en diez a una en veinte casos.
Q. (Dad): If this occurs, what do you do?	(Papá): Si esto sucede, ¿qué van a hacer?	(Papá): ¿Qué hacen en ese caso?
A. We remove the stitches and let the infection drain out and let the wound heal in from the bottom (secondary intention).	Le quitamos las costuras y dejamos que la infección drene y que la herida se cure desde el fondo.	Le quitamos las suturas y dejamos que la infección se seque y que la herida se cure desde el fondo.
Q. For pain, Tom, you can take Tylenol or ibuprofen. Take the ibuprofen with food otherwise it can irritate your stomach. No playing sports until we see you back and get the sutures out. Do either of you have any other questions?	Tom, para el dolor puedes tomar Tylenol o Ibuprofen. El Ibuprofen tiene que tomarlo con comida para que no le irrite el estómago. No debe jugar deportes hasta que lo veamos otra vez y le quitemos las costuras. ¿Alguno tiene preguntas?	Tom puede tomar Tylenol o Ibuprofen para el dolor. El Ibuprofen hay que tomarlo con comida para que no le moleste al estómago. No debe jugar deportes hasta que lo veamos otra vez y le quitemos las suturas. ¿Tiene preguntas?
A. No, Doctor, we will see you in a week.	No, doctora. La veremos en una semana.	No, doctora, nos vemos la próxima semana.

CASE 5: ABNORMAL DEVELOPMENT

The final case is not what might be considered an emergency but is a common complaint heard by clinicians who see children in their practices. Frequently, parents are concerned over the motor or cognitive development of their children. The truth is that there is tremendous variation in childhood development. True, we are taught developmental landmarks, but these represent the mean. For example, most children will speak their first word by 12 months old, but there are some who do not speak until later, yet are very normal in their subsequent development. However, if a landmark such as sitting up, walking, smiling, or language is delayed, we have to be concerned that maybe there is some problem. The following are general developmental landmarks.

DEVELOPMENTAL LANDMARKS

Motor	Cognitive
Holding head up prone: 0–3 months	Smiling socially: 1–3 months
Turning over: 3–6 months	Saying first word: 6–12 months
Crawling: 6–12 months	
Sitting up: 4–8 months	
Walking: 8–15 months	

Later on, problems—especially cognitive ones—will come up at school, such as doing poorly in class, etc. There are many causes for this, ranging from hearing problems resulting from recurrent ear infections to drug or alcohol problems. Often the cause is problems within the family.

HISTORY OF PRESENT ILLNESS

Maria is a 5-year-old girl who is having problems in class. She still is not able to read the letters of the alphabet and her comprehension of spoken words is very delayed according to her teacher and her mother. Her motor development appears normal.

	English	Spanish Formal	Spanish Informal
Q.	Good morning, Ms. Soto. Good morning, Maria. I am Doctor Brown. What brings you to see us today?	Buenos días, Srta. Soto. Buenos días, María. Soy el doctor Brown. ¿Por qué viene a vernos el día de hoy?	Buenos días, Srta. Soto. Buenos días, María. Soy el doctor Brown. ¿Por qué vino hoy?
A.	Good morning, Doctor, my daughter Maria is having problems in school. She started kindergarten and the teacher says she isn't learning like the other kids. I have three other children who are older and they all spoke much earlier and better than Maria. She also has a hard time understanding me.	Buenos días, doctor, mi hija María está teniendo problemas en la escuela. Comenzó en el jardín infantil y la maestra dice que no está aprendiendo como los otros niños. Tengo tres niños más que son mayorcitos y todos empezaron a hablar más temprano y mejor que María. También le cuesta mucho entenderme.	Buenos días, doctor. María, mi hija, tiene problemas en la escuela. Comenzó en el jardín infantil y la maestra dice que no está aprendiendo igual que los otros niños. Tengo tres más que son mayorcitos y todos comenzaron a hablar más temprano y mejor que María. También no me entiende nada.
Q.	Is she able to run and play like the other children?	¿Puede correr y jugar como las otras niñas?	¿Corre y juega como las otras niñas?
A.	She is doing well in that part of her development. She runs and plays with her brothers and sisters normally.	Está bien en esa parte de su desarrollo. Corre y juega con sus hermanos y hermanas normalmente.	No tiene problemas en esa parte del desarrollo. Corre y juega con sus hermanos y hermanas todo el tiempo.

	English	Spanish Formal	Spanish Informal Continued
Q.	Were her birth and delivery normal or were there complications such as premature delivery or problems with the delivery?	¿Tuvo un nacimiento y parto normales o hubo complicaciones, como parto prematuro o problemas del parto?	¿El nacimiento y parto fueron normales o hubo complicaciones, como parto prematuro o problemas para nacer?
A.	She was one month premature.	Fue prematura por un mes.	Nació un mes antes.
Q.	How much did she weigh?	¿Cuánto pesó al nacer?	¿Cuánto pesó?
A.	She weighed 4 pounds 12 ounces.	Pesó cuatro libras y doce onzas.	Cuatro libras y doce onzas.
Q.	Did she have breathing problems at birth such as requiring oxygen?	¿Tuvo problemas para respirar al nacer? ¿Le tuvieron que poner oxígeno?	¿Tuvo problemas para respirar cuando nació? ¿Le pusieron oxígeno?
A.	Yes, she required oxygen for about a week.	Sí, estuvo con oxígeno por una semana.	Sí, le pusieron oxígeno por una semana.
Q.	Did she require a breathing tube and machine to help her breathe? Was she in the intensive care unit after her birth?	¿Le tuvieron que poner un tubo y conectarla a una máquina para que pudiera respirar? ¿Estuvo internada en la unidad de cuidados intensivos después de nacer?	¿Le pusieron un tubo y la conectaron a una máquina para respirar?
A.	She was there for about two or three days.	Estuvo internada ahí como dos o tres días.	Estuvo en la unidad de cuidados intensivos. Estuvo ahí como dos o tres días.
Q.	Did her skin turn yellow after birth?	¿Se le puso amarilla la piel después de nacer?	Después de nacer, ¿se le puso amarilla la piel?
A.	Yes. About two days after she was born she became yellow.	Sí. Como dos días después de nacer, se le puso la piel amarilla.	Sí. Se puso amarilla como dos días después de nacer.
Q.	What did they do for this?	¿Qué le hicieron para ese problema?	¿Qué le hicieron?
A.	They put her under some lights for about three days and it went away.	La pusieron debajo de un tipo de luz por tres días y se le quitó.	Le pusieron bajo la luz por tres días y se le quitó.
Q.	Did she have seizures at birth or in the hospital after?	¿Tuvo convulsiones cuando nació o en el hospital, después?	¿Padeció de convulsiones al nacer o después, en el hospital?
A.	She has never had convulsions.	Nunca ha tenido convulsiones.	No.
Q.	How long did she remain in the hospital?	¿Cuánto tiempo estuvo internada en el hospital?	¿Cuánto tiempo estuvo en el hospital?
A.	She stayed one week.	Estuvo internada una semana.	Una semana.

The birth history is a critical part of the questioning in a child who has had motor or cognitive delay. Whether the baby was term (i.e., 40 weeks) at the time of birth and birth weight are important questions. In premature babies, often the lungs are not completely developed and oxygen exchange is impaired. Hypoxemia at birth may result in brain damage, especially if not treated promptly. A traumatic birth such as occurs with meconium aspiration, a condition where the newborn aspirates the stomach contents resulting in pneumonia, may produce hypoxemia in a full term baby, resulting in brain damage. Thus, the birth history is important in this patient. Jaundice in the premature newborn is common due in most cases to an immature liver enzyme system used to degrade bilirubin. If the levels of bilirubin get too high, however, permanent brain damage may occur due to the permeability in the infant of the blood-brain barrier to bilirubin, which can deposit in the brain and cause permanent damage, a disease termed kernicterus. This blood-brain barrier becomes impermeable to bilirubin by age. Finally, seizures in the newborn are a grave sign always indicating some pathologic condition. Infection such as meningitis can result in seizures, as can hypoxemia, underlying hemorrhage, and hypoglycemia. Unfortunately, seizures in the newborn carry a poor prognosis in terms of later development.

	English	Spanish Formal	Spanish Informal
Q.	Since birth during the first year of life did she gain weight normally?	¿Ganó peso normalmente durante el primer año de vida, desde que nació?	¿Aumentó de peso normalmente en el primer año de vida?
A.	Yes she gained weight rapidly. The pediatrician said she was normal weight and height.	Sí, ganó peso rápidamente. El pediatra me dijo que el peso y la talla eran normales.	Sí, el pediatra me dijo que el peso y la talla eran normales.
Q.	When did she sit up?	¿A qué edad se sentó por primera vez?	¿Qué edad tenía cuando se sentó?
A.	Around three months.	Como tres meses.	Tres meses.
Q.	When did she start to crawl?	¿A qué edad empezó a gatear?	¿Cuándo comenzó a gatear?
A.	At about six months.	Como a los seis meses.	A los seis.
Q.	When did she stand and when did she first walk?	¿A qué edad se puso de pie y cuándo comenzó a caminar?	¿Cuándo se puso de pie y cuándo empezó a caminar?
A.	I don't know when she first stood but she walked at about one year.	No me acuerdo cuándo se puso de pie la primera vez, pero comenzó a caminar cuando tenía un año.	Empezó a caminar cuando tenía un año, pero no recuerdo cuándo se puso de pie la primera vez.
Q.	When did she say her first words?	¿A qué edad dijo las primeras palabras?	¿Cuándo comenzó a decir las primeras palabras?
A.	She was about one year old when she said her first words.	Tenía como un año de edad cuando dijo sus primeras palabras.	Cuando tenía como un año.
Q.	When did she start speaking in sentences?	¿A qué edad comenzó a hablar en oraciones?	¿Cuándo comenzó a decir frases enteras?
A.	At about three years of age.	Como a los tres años.	Cuando tenía tres años.
Q.	Does Maria use diapers or can she use the toilet?	¿María usa pañales o ya puede ir al servicio sanitario?	¿María usa pañales o ya puede ir al excusado?
A.	She usually uses the toilet but she still wets her bed occasionally at night.	Generalmente usa el servicio, pero de vez en cuando todavía se orina en la cama en la noche.	Ya usa el excusado, pero a veces en la noche todavía se orina en la cama.
Q.	What grade is Maria in now?	¿En qué año de la escuela está María ahora?	En la escuela, ¿en qué año está?
A.	She is in kindergarten.	Está en el jardín infantil.	Está en el kinder.
Q.	How is she doing in school now in regard to writing and reading?	¿Cómo le va con la lectura y la escritura en la escuela ahora?	¿Tiene problemas para leer o escribir en la escuela?
A.	The teacher says she is having problems writing her alphabet. She still can't read any words. She also has trouble understanding in class when she is asked to do a task.	El maestro dice que tiene problemas escribiendo las letras del alfabeto. Todavía no puede leer ninguna palabra. También tiene dificultad para entender en clase cuando le piden que complete alguna tarea.	Tiene problemas escribiendo las letras del alfabeto. No puede leer ninguna palabra todavía. Y le cuesta entender en clase cuando le dicen que haga algún ejercicio.

	English	Spanish Formal	Spanish Informal	Continued
Q.	At home do you read with her and work with her on the alphabet?	¿Usted le lee y la ayuda a trabajar con el alfabeto en la casa?	¿En la casa usted lee con ella y le ayuda a trabajar con el alfabeto?	
A.	Yes. Every night I read books to her recommended by her teacher and I try to get her to write her alphabet, but it is a struggle for her.	Sí. Todas las noches le leo libros que le recomienda la maestra y trato de que escriba el alfabeto, pero le cuesta mucho.	Sí. Le leo libros que le recomienda la maestra todas las noches y trato de que escriba el alfabeto, pero es muy difícil para ella.	
Q.	Has Maria had episodes of ear infections in the past?	¿Alguna vez María ha tenido episodios de infecciones en el oído?	¿María padece de infecciones en el oído?	
A.	She had one ear infection when she was three but that is the only one.	Tuvo una infección en el oído cuando tenía tres años, pero esa fue la única vez.	Cuando tenía tres años, tuvo una infección en el oído, pero esa fue la única vez.	
Q.	Does she hear you okay when you talk to her or does it appear that she has trouble hearing?	¿La escucha bien cuando usted le habla o parece que tiene dificultad para escuchar?	¿La oye bien cuando usted le habla o parece que le cuesta oír?	
A.	No, she hears okay I think because when I ask her questions in a simple way she can answer me. She can also hear the dog bark when he wants to come in the house.	No, yo creo que escucha bien porque cuando le hago preguntas sencillas, me contesta. También puede escuchar el perro ladrando cuando quiere entrar en la casa.	No, yo pienso que oye bien porque cuando le hago preguntas sencillas, me contesta. También puede oír el perro ladrando cuando quiere meterse en la casa.	
Q.	Do you think she sees normally?	¿Usted cree que puede ver normalmente?	¿Usted piensa que está bien de la vista?	
A.	Yes I believe so. She had her vision tested a month ago because of the concern over her difficulty in school.	Yo creo que sí. Le hicieron una prueba de la vista hace un mes porque estábamos preocupados por la dificultad que tiene en la escuela.	Creo que sí. Le hicieron un examen hace un mes porque estábamos preocupados por los problemas que tiene en la escuela.	
Q.	Does Maria have any brothers or sisters? If so, are they doing well in school?	¿María tiene hermanos o hermanas? ¿Les va bien en la escuela?	¿Tiene María hermanos o hermanas? ¿Y les va bien en la escuela?	
A.	She has a brother and sister both older than her and they are both doing very well in school.	Tiene un hermano y una hermana. Los dos son mayores que ella y les va muy bien en la escuela.	Sí, tiene un hermano y una hermana. Ambos son mayores que ella y les va muy bien en la escuela.	
Q.	Ms. Soto, I need to do a physical exam. It will make it easier for Maria if you can remain in the room.	Srta. Soto, necesito hacer un examen físico. Si usted se queda en el cuarto, va a ser más fácil para María.	Srta. Soto, tengo que hacer un examen físico. Va a ser más fácil para María si usted se queda en el cuarto.	
A.	That's fine.	Está bien.	Bien.	

PHYSICAL EXAM

In a five-year-old with a delay in development, a complete physical exam should be done. This includes the usual listening to the heart and lungs, examining the head and neck region with careful attention to the ear exam. As noted above, ear infections can result in a hearing loss, causing problems with learning. In this case, you might note scarring of the tympanic membranes or fluid behind the membrane. The eye exam is likewise important, including the fundoscopic exam to visualize the retina and the optic disc. Of main concern here is the neurologic exam. Checking the motor exam and cognitive function, one has to be creative. Using a stuffed animal to assess gross motor movement is helpful, and color cards when testing recognition of different objects and animals is helpful. Here the clinician is testing gross motor function as well as cognitive function. The purpose of the exam is to support the history of a delay in development and at times one might even discover the cause, as in the case of inner ear pathology. Often, as in this case, a referral is made to a pediatric neurologist and psychologist for sophisticated testing to further clarify the problem.

FOLLOW-UP

	English	Spanish Formal	Spanish Informal
Q.	Ms. Soto, based on what you have told me and based on our brief exam, I feel your daughter should be referred for further testing to a pediatric psychologist and neurologist. It may be that the problem comes from her premature birth. It is not uncommon to see some problems as children enter school. Sometimes with special techniques children can advance rapidly to where they should be. Other times it is a slower process. I will make the referrals now. Do you have any questions?	Srta. Soto. De acuerdo con lo que usted me dijo y con el examen que le hicimos, yo pienso que su hija debería ser referida a un pediatra psicólogo y a un neurólogo para que le hagan otros exámenes. Es posible que el problema venga de su nacimiento prematuro. No es raro ver algunos problemas cuando los niños entran a la escuela. A veces, con técnicas especiales, los niños pueden avanzar rápidamente a donde deben estar. Otras veces, es un proceso lento. Voy a hacer la referencia ahora. ¿Tiene alguna pregunta?	Srta. Soto. De acuerdo con lo que usted me dijo y el examen, yo creo que hay que mandar a su hija para que la vea un pediatra psicólogo y un neurólogo y le hagan exámenes adicionales. Puede ser que el problema venga del nacimiento prematuro. No es raro ver estos problemas cuando los niños entran a la escuela. A veces, con técnicas especiales, pueden avanzar rápidamente a donde deben estar. Otras veces, es más lento. Voy a hacer la referencia ahora. ¿Tiene preguntas?
A.	Do you think she will be "slow" the rest of her life?	¿Usted piensa que va a ser "lenta" el resto de su vida?	¿Usted cree que va a ser "lerdita" el resto de su vida?
Q.	It is not uncommon that children advance at different rates in school regardless of their intelligence. It is difficult to say at this age if this is due to a neurologic problem—for example, some brain injury at birth—or if this is just that children advance at different rates. For that reason it is important to come up with the reason for Maria's problems in school. The specialists we are referring her to will make this determination. It is important to define the cause of the problem because there are different techniques to assure that Maria will get the best possible education.	No es raro que los niños avancen a un paso diferente en la escuela a pesar de ser inteligentes. Es difícil decir a esta edad si se debe a problemas neurológicos, como por ejemplo una lesión cerebral al nacer, o si es sólo que todos los niños avanzan a un paso diferente. Por esa razón, es importante averiguar la causa de los problemas que María tiene en la escuela. Los especialistas donde la vamos a referir tienen que hacer esta determinación. Es importante definir la causa del problema porque hay diferentes técnicas para asegurar que María reciba acute; la mejor educación posible.	Es común que los niños progresen a un paso diferente en la escuela, aunque sean inteligentes. Es difícil decir a esta edad si es por problemas neurológicos, como una lesión cerebral al nacer, o si es sólo que cada niño progresa a un paso diferente. Por eso es que es importante saber la causa de los problemas que María tiene en la escuela. Los especialistas donde la vamos a mandar tienen que decidir. Es importante saber la causa del problema porque hay diferentes técnicas para asegurar que María reciba la mejor educación posible.
A.	Thank you!	¡Gracias!	¡Muchas gracias!

There is nothing more frightening to a parent than this situation. Imagine the thoughts that go through a parent's head. It is crucial that this child receives a correct diagnosis; her future will depend on it. As a general pediatrician or family physician, the original screening is crucial to identify who should be referred to a specialist versus the majority of children who have problems in school due to other reasons that can be managed by the primary care physician.

Although we have covered a limited number of specific diseases, by being creative with the Spanish language you can cover most clinical scenarios by using the format in the above dialogues. For example, a child who presents with suspected pneumonia or asthma. The key is to keep things as simple as possible. Try to keep your sentences concise. If you don't understand an answer, you can say "*¿Qué quiere decir?*" i.e., What do you mean? and your patient will re-phrase the answer. If they speak too fast, you can ask them to slow down, "*¿Puede hablar más despacio, por favor?*" i.e., Can you speak slower, please? These are some of the approaches you can use to better understand your patients.

VOCABULARY

English	Español
Appetite	Apetito, hambre
Asthma	Asma, apretazón de pecho, ahogo
Blood test	Prueba de sangre
Bronchitis	Bronquitis
Bruise	Moretón
Chest	Pecho, tórax
Cold	Resfrío, gripe
Colic	Cólico, retortijón
Contagious	Contagioso, se pega
Cough	Tos
Culture	Cultivo
Dehydrated	Deshidratado
Diabetes	Diabetes
Ear	Oreja
Ear, inner ear	Oído
Earache	Dolor de oído
Fever	Fiebre, calentura
Flu	Gripe, catarro
Gastroenteritis	Gastroenteritis, mal de estómago, obradera
Headache	Dolor de cabeza
Hepatitis	Hepatitis, amarillón
Infection	Infección
Itch	Comezón, picazón, rasquera
Lungs	Pulmones
Lymph nodes	Ganglios linfáticos, nódulos linfáticos
Measles	Sarampión
Meningitis	Meningitis
Mumps	Paperas

English	Español
Neck	Cuello, pescuezo
Nose	Nariz
Pale	Pálido, blanco como el papel
Phlegm	Flema, gargajo
Pneumonia	Neumonía, pulmonía
Rash	Sarpullido, mancha, salpullido
Rubella	Rubéola
Scabies	Sarna, rasquiña
Scratch	Rasguño
Short of breath	Falta de aire, falta de respiración, dificultad para respirar
Sore throat	Dolor de garganta, infección de la garganta
Spinal tap	Punción lumbar
Tetanus	Tétano
Throat	Garganta
Tired	Cansado, agotado
To lose weight	Bajar de peso, perder peso, perder libras
To pull	Halar, tirar, jalar
To urinate	Orinar
Tonsils	Amígdalas, anginas, glándulas
Urine analysis	Examen de orina
Urine sample	Muestra de orina
Vomit	Vómito
X-rays	Rayos X, radiografía

GRAMMATICAL TIPS

PRETERITE TENSE

When asking questions in a clinical history or gathering information about the patient, the provider will be using the preterite tense and the imperfect tense to interrogate the patient. The preterite is used with single completed events in the past, for example, when asking about when a symptom started, when it ended, how many times it happened, etc. These past actions have been completed as facts. There is a specific time frame.

The conjugation for the regular verbs in the preterite is as follows. Verbs ending in:

-ar	-er	-ir
Hablar	Comer	Vivir
Hablé	Comí	Viví
Hablaste	Comiste	Viviste
Habló	Comió	Vivió
Hablamos	Comimos	Vivimos
Hablaron	Comieron	Vivieron

Stem-Changing Verbs

For these types of verbs, there are three rules that must be met. Only stem-changing verbs that end in *ir* in the present can be stem-changing in the *pretérito*. There are only two stem changes: *e-i* and *o-u*. And only the third person changes the stem.

Examples:

Repetir	Dormir
Repetí	Dormí
Repetiste	Dormiste
Repitió	Durmió
Repetimos	Dormimos
Repitieron	Durmieron

Spelling-Changing Verbs

These verbs change their spelling because of phonetics—sound overrides grammar rules. Examples are verbs that end in *uir* or *eer* such as *construir* (to build), *huir* (to run away), *leer* (to read), or *creer* (to believe). They change the third person:

Construí	Creí
Construiste	Creiste
Construyó	Creyó
Construimos	Creimos
Construyeron	Creyeron

Other verbs that change their spelling are verbs that end in *car*, *gar*, and *zar*. Again, these verbs change their spelling because there are no words with syllables *ze* or *zi* in Spanish. These verbs only change their spelling in the *yo* form since it is the only ending that has an *e* or *i*.

Buscar = busqué	Cargar = cargué	Empezar = empecé

Irregular Verbs

Irregular verbs do not follow any rules. These verbs are the hardest verbs to remember. They have been categorized by endings and the changes in their stems as i group, u group, and pure irregulars. The endings are as follows:

- -e i verbs u group verbs j group verbs
- -iste
- -o
- -imos
- -ieron

IMPERFECT TENSE

It is used when stating thoughts in the past that are not time-specific. When asking repeated, habitual actions in the past, we use the imperfect. Imperfect is also used for actions that might still be present. In general, the imperfect does not necessarily care about time, when something started or when it ended. It fluctuates through time and space.

Imperfect conjugations:

-ar	-er	-ir
Hablar	Comer	Vivir
Hablaba	Comía	Vivía
Hablabas	Comías	Vivías
Hablaba	Comía	Vivía
Hablábamos	Comíamos	Vivíamos
Hablaban	Comían	Vivían

There are only three irregular verbs in the imperfect:

Ir	Ser	Ver
Iba	Era	Veía
Ibas	Eras	Veías
Iba	Era	Veía
Íbamos	Éramos	Veíamos
Iban	Eran	Veían

Ejercicios Sobre el Pretérito:

Please conjugate the following verbs in the preterite:

El doctor _____ (*decir*) que tengo que hacer ejercicio regularmente.

Yo _____ (*seguir*) las instrucciones al pie de la letra.

Cuando _____ (*ir*) a la cita, el médico me _____ (*confirmar*) la sospecha: ¡estoy embarazada!

Cuéntame lo que te _____ (*pasar*) en el consultorio, me _____ (llamar, tú), y tu padre y yo nos _____ (*quedar*) preocupados.

Disculpe, señora, pero la cita de sus hijos con el doctor Martínez se _____ (*cancelar*) ayer.

Ejercicios Sobre el Imperfecto:

Please conjugate the following verbs in the imperfect:

Mientras la enfermera me _____ (*tomar*) la presión arterial, la gente _____ (*caminar*) y no _____ (*poder, ella*) escuchar el estetoscopio.

Cuando _____ (*trabajar*) en el hospital, yo _____ (*interpretar*) para los pacientes que no _____ (*hablar*) inglés.

_____ (*ser*) las diez de la noche y no _____ (*haber*) personal en la sala de emergencias.

There are some verbs that change their meanings when they are used in the preterite:

	Imperfect	Preterite
Querer (To want)	Quería (Wanted)	Quise (I tried and failed)
No querer (Not to want)	No quería (Did not want)	No quise (Refused)
Saber (To know)	Sabía (Knew)	Supe (I found out)
Conocer (To know)	Conocía (Used to know)	Conocí (I met)
Poder (To be able to)	Podía (Was able to)	Pude (I tried and succeeded)
No poder (Not to be able to)	No podía (Was not able to)	No pude (I tried and failed)
Tener (To have)	Tenía (Used to have)	Tuve (Got or received)

Ejercicios con el pretérito y el imperfecto:

Please decide whether the *pretérito* or the *imperfecto* will be used in the following sentences, and conjugate the verbs:

Ayer que _____ (*estudiar*) para el examen de la clase, me _____ (*sentir*) preparada.

Cuando el paciente _____ (*entrar*) a la clínica, _____ (*saber*) que el doctor lo _____ (*esperar*)

Al momento que lo _____ (*ver*), _____ (*saber*), que el diagnóstico _____ (*ser*) positivo.

An option not to use the *pretérito* altogether: when an action started in the past and still is occurring in the present, present perfect can be used. A commonly used form in questioning a patient is *Ha tenido . . .* such as in *¿Ha tenido dolor?* (= Have you had pain?). This is called the present perfect tense. It is a very useful and simple verb form to use when asking your patient questions. To form the present perfect in Spanish, you need the present conjugation of the verb *haber; he, has, ha, hemos, han,* and the past participle of the main verb. The *er* ending of the verb *tener* is dropped and *ido* is added.

For example:

Tener: ¿Ha tenido fiebre? (= Have you had fever?)
Comer: ¿Ha comido hoy? (= Have you eaten today?)
Mover: ¿Ha movido la pierna? (= Have you moved the leg?)

For verbs ending in *ar* such as *tomar* or *cambiar,* drop *ar* and add *ado.* The conjugation of the auxiliary verb *haber* remains exactly the same. For example:

Tomar: ¿Ha tomado algún medicamento? (= Have you taken any medicine?)
Cambiar: ¿Ha cambiado el dolor? (= Has the pain changed?)
Vomitar: ¿Ha vomitado desde ayer? (= Have you vomited since yesterday?)

And for verbs ending in *ir* such as *vivir,* drop *ir* and add *ido.* Although there are some irregular verbs that don't follow this rule, the verbs usually used in conversing with your patient do.

Tener	**Tomar**
Yo he tenido = I have had	*Yo he tomado* = I have drunk
Tú has tenido = You have had	*Tú has tomado* = You have drunk
Ella, Él, Usted ha tenido = He or she has had	*Ella, Él, Usted ha tomado* = He or she has drunk

The following examples are with the verb *tener* and *ir* in the preterite. The conjugation is irregular since the verb tener is one of those u group verbs and *ir* has the same conjugation as that of *ser*.

Ayer tuve dolor. (= I had pain yesterday)
Ayer fui al médico. (= I went to the doctor's yesterday)

Tener	**Ir**
Yo tuve = I had	*Yo fui* = I went
Tú tuviste = You had	*Tú fuiste* = You went
Ella, Él, Usted tuvo = He or she had	*Ella, Él, Usted fue* = He or she went

The imperfect form of the past tense is used with repeated or habitual actions. When an incident or action is continuous and unfinished, for example:

María tenía mucha fiebre por la noche. (= Maria had a lot of fever during the night.)

The imperfect tense of regular verbs in Spanish is formed with the root or stem plus particular endings. The stem is formed by dropping *ar*, *er*, or *ir*. For example:

Tener	Tomar	Vivir
Yo tenía = I had	*Yo tomaba* = I drank	*Yo vivía* = I lived
Tú tenías = You had	*Tú tomabas* = You drank	*Tú vivías* = You lived
Ella, Él, Usted tenía = He or she had	*Ella, Él, Usted tomaba* = He or she drank	*Ella, Él, Usted vivía* = He or she lived

CULTURAL TIPS: CURANDERISMO

Curanderismo, or shamanism, is a traditional form of alternative medicine. The *curandero* or shaman plays an essential role in various communities. There are areas in Latin America where people will go first to a *curandero* and then to a doctor if they have access to one. Usually the curandero treats illnesses in different ways. The belief is that most of the illnesses have a spiritual and energy foundation and therefore a *limpia,* or a cleansing, is necessary. After this is done, the illness is cured. When the illness does not improve, the options vary and herbs or massages can be used. Different remedies have been found to be effective in treating certain illnesses. In the United States, there have been conferences with curanderos and people who are interested in learning about this form of medicine. Some states have hosted such conferences with successful results. The ways of selecting illnesses vary. It is believed that the body needs to be in balance. There is a binary of cold/hot and wet/dry. If there is an illness produced by an imbalance, then there is a need to find equilibrium in the body.

4 Gynecologic Diseases

INTRODUCTION

ANATOMY

The basic anatomy of the female reproductive tract is depicted in Figure 4-1.

DISEASE CATEGORIES

As we have done in the preceding chapters, it is important when seeing a patient with a gynecologic disease to think in terms of emergent, urgent, and non-urgent categories. Included in the emergent presentations is ectopic pregnancy, which is a life-threatening problem in a woman of childbearing age. Undiagnosed, the woman may exsanguinate, thus this disease always has to be included in the differential diagnosis when a woman of childbearing age presents with abdominal pain and/or "spotting" (discharge of blood per vagina)

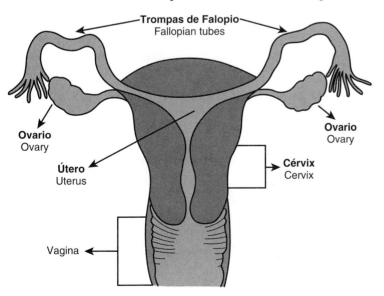

Figure 4-1. Anatomy of the female reproductive system in English and Spanish.

Trompas de Falopio
Fallopian tubes

Ovario
Ovary

Ovario
Ovary

Útero
Uterus

Cérvix
Cervix

Vagina

in between menstrual periods. Urgent diseases include pelvic inflammatory disease (PID), which is an infection in the fallopian tubes caused by bacterial infection and usually transmitted sexually. Also included in the urgent category would be vaginal bleeding in a woman who is post-menopausal, which might be the presentation of endometrial cancer. This patient may not need admission to the hospital, but a prompt workup to exclude the diagnosis of uterine cancer is warranted. Chronic or non-urgent disease states may include heavy or irregular menstrual periods, infertility problems, and chronic abdominal pain from endometriosis, which often are of great concern but can be managed on an outpatient basis. We will illustrate in the cases presented below one case from each category.

CASE 1: ECTOPIC PREGNANCY

CHIEF COMPLAINT

Ms. Padilla, a 22-year-old woman, presents to your clinic with lower abdominal pain. Her **vital signs** are as follows: Temp. 37° C, P 64, BP 120/62.

HISTORY

	English	Spanish Formal	Spanish Informal
Q.	Hello, Ms. Padilla. My name is Dr. Marcelo. What brings you to see us today?	Hola, Srta. Padilla. Soy el Dr. Marcelo. ¿Por qué viene a vernos hoy?	Hola, Srta. Padilla. Soy el Dr. Marcelo. ¿Qué molestias tiene?
A.	I have had pain in my stomach for the past day.	He tenido dolor de estómago todo el día.	Me ha dolido el estómago todo el día.
Q.	How old are you?	¿Qué edad tiene?	¿Cuántos años tiene?
A.	I am 22 years old.	Tengo veintidós años de edad.	Veintidós años.
Q.	Where is it located?	¿Dónde es el dolor?	¿Dónde le duele?
A.	In the lower part, more on the right side.	En la parte de abajo, más hacia la derecha.	Aquí, en la parte de abajo, a la derecha.
Q.	When did it start?	¿Cuándo le comenzó?	¿Cuándo empezó?
A.	It started yesterday morning and the pain is much worse now.	El dolor me comenzó ayer por la mañana y es peor ahora.	Empezó ayer en la mañana y es peor hoy.
Q.	What makes it better or worse?	¿Qué mejora o empeora el dolor?	¿Qué lo hace mejor o peor?
A.	When I move around it is much worse than when I lie down and don't move.	Cuando me muevo es peor que cuando me acuesto y me quedo quieta (no me muevo).	Cuando me muevo es peor. Cuando estoy quieta, es mejor.
Q.	How would you describe the pain? For example, is it sharp or dull?	¿Cómo describiría el dolor? Por ejemplo, ¿es sordo o punzante (agudo)?	¿Cómo es el dolor? ¿Es agudo, punzante o sordo?
A.	It is sharp now but at the beginning it was dull.	Es punzante (agudo) ahora, pero al principio era sordo (por todos lados, por todo el estómago).	Al principio era sordo, pero ahora es punzante (agudo).

English	Spanish Formal	Spanish Informal
Q. On a scale of one to ten, ten being the worst, how would you grade the pain?	En una escala de uno a diez, donde diez es el peor dolor que usted ha tenido en su vida, ¿cómo catalogaría (clasificaría) este dolor?	De uno a diez, donde diez es el peor dolor que ha tenido, ¿cómo diría usted que es este dolor?
A. It is about a seven.	Es como un siete.	Un siete.
Q. Is the pain constant, or does it come and go?	¿El dolor es constante o le va y le viene?	¿Le pega y se le quita o lo tiene todo el tiempo?
A. The pain is constant.	El dolor es constante.	Todo el tiempo.
Q. Does it move anywhere or does it stay in one spot?	¿Se mueve a algún lugar o se queda en el mismo sitio?	¿Se le mueve para algún otro lugar?
A. It stays in one area, the lower right side of my stomach.	Se queda en la misma área (lugar), el lado de abajo y derecho del estómago.	Se queda en el mismo lugar. Debajo del estómago y a la derecha.
Q. Are there any other symptoms that you have, such as fever, chills, nausea, vomiting, or diarrhea?	¿Tiene algún otro síntoma, como fiebre, escalofríos, nausea, vómitos o diarrea?	¿Tiene otros síntomas, como ganas de vomitar, escalofríos o diarrea?
A. I have had some nausea and vomited once. I haven't taken my temperature but I have felt normal. I have had no chills or diarrhea.	He tenido un poco de náusea y vomité una vez. No me he tomado la temperatura, pero me he sentido normal. No he tenido diarrea ni escalofríos.	Ganas de vomitar. Vomité una vez.
Q. When was your last period and was it normal?	¿Cuándo fue su última regla (menstruación)? ¿Era normal?	¿Cuándo tuvo usted la última regla? ¿Fue normal?
A. It was one month ago and it was normal.	Fue hace un mes y me vino normal.	Hace un mes. Y fue normal.
Q. Have you ever been pregnant before?	¿Alguna vez ha estado embarazada?	¿Ha estado embarazada?
A. No, never.	No, nunca.	No.
Q. Have you had any "spotting" or abnormal vaginal bleeding since your last period?	¿Ha tenido algún "manchado" o sangrado anormal por la vagina desde que tuvo la última regla?	Después de la regla, ¿ha tenido algún sangrado o manchado?
A. No, I have had no bleeding.	No, no he tenido ningún sangrado.	No.
Q. Do you have any vaginal discharge?	¿Tiene algún flujo (desecho, secreción) vaginal?	¿Tiene desecho?
A. No, not that I have noted.	No, no que yo haya notado.	No.
Q. Are you active sexually and do you use some form of birth control?	¿Está teniendo relaciones sexuales? ¿Usa algún método anticonceptivo (para prevenir el embarazo)?	¿Tiene relaciones sexuales? ¿Usa algún método para evitar el embarazo?
A. Yes, I am active sexually and my boyfriend and I use protection (condoms); however, lately we haven't been that good about remembering.	Sí, tengo relaciones sexuales con mi novio, y él y yo usamos protección (condones); pero últimamente no nos hemos acordado.	Sí, con mi novio. A veces usamos condones y a veces no.
Q. Is there any chance that you are pregnant?	¿Hay alguna posibilidad de que usted esté embarazada?	¿Usted cree que puede estar embarazada?
A. There is a possibility.	Es posible.	Tal vez.

	English	Spanish Formal	Spanish Informal Continued
Q.	Have you felt sick to your stomach in the morning or noted that your breasts feel swollen?	¿Ha sentido ganas de vomitar por la mañana? O ¿ha notado que tiene los senos hinchados *(siente hinchazón en el busto)*?	¿Ha tenido ganas de vomitar en la mañana o notado que tiene el busto inflamado?
A.	I have had some nausea in the morning lately. My breasts do feel swollen.	Últimamente he tenido ganas de vomitar por la mañana. Siento los senos hinchados.	Sí, he estado con ganas de vomitar en la mañana y siento el busto un poco hinchado.
Q.	Have you ever had an infection in your vagina, uterus, or tubes where they had to give you antibiotics?	¿Alguna vez ha tenido una infección en la vagina, el útero o las trompas de Falopio, para la que tuvieron que darle antibióticos?	¿Ha tenido una infección en los genitales *(la vagina, la matriz)*? ¿Le dieron antibióticos?
A.	No, I have had no infections in those parts.	No, no he tenido infecciones en esas partes.	No.
Q.	Have you felt lightheaded or dizzy lately?	¿Alguna vez en los últimos días se ha sentido débil o mareada?	¿Ha tenido mareos o se ha sentido débil?
A.	I have felt very tired lately.	Últimamente me he sentido muy cansada.	Me he sentido muy cansada.
Q.	Are you otherwise in good health? Do you have any heart, lung, or stomach problems?	Aparte de esto, ¿tiene *(usted)* algún otro problema de salud? ¿Tiene algún problema del corazón, los pulmones o el estómago?	¿Padece del corazón, los pulmones, el estómago u otra cosa?
A.	I have asthma but haven't had to take medicines since I was a child.	Tengo asma, pero no he tenido que tomar medicinas desde que era niña.	De asma, pero no he tomado medicinas desde pequeñita.
Q.	Are you taking any medications, including non-prescription medications?	¿Está tomando alguna medicina, incluyendo medicinas sin receta o de la yerbería *(botica)*?	¿Toma alguna medicina de la farmacia o de la curandera?
A.	Just ibuprofen for headache once in a while.	Sólo ibuprofen de vez en cuando para los dolores de cabeza.	Ibuprofen para el dolor de la cabeza de vez en cuando.
Q.	Do you have any allergy to medications?	¿Padece de alergia a alguna medicina?	¿Es alérgica a alguna medicina?
A.	I am allergic to penicillin.	Soy alérgica a la penicilina.	Tengo alergia a la penicilina.
Q.	What happened when you took it?	¿Qué pasó cuando la tomó la última vez?	¿Qué pasa cuando toma penicilina?
A.	I broke out in a rash.	Me broté en *(me salió)* un sarpullido *(salpullido, una mancha)*.	Me broto en un sarpullido por todo el cuerpo.
	Ms. Padilla, we are going to go ahead and do a physical exam including a pelvic exam. While you are changing into a gown, we are going to go ahead and have blood drawn to see if you are pregnant and check your blood count. We will also perform an ultrasound exam of your stomach. There is a possibility that you are pregnant. If that turns out to be the case, we need to check and make sure the baby is in the right place. Sometimes the baby can be in the tube instead of the uterus. The ultrasound will tell us that. Can you please change into a gown? I will return with one of the nurses in a few minutes to do the exam.	Srta. Padilla, le vamos a hacer un examen físico, incluyendo un examen de la pelvis *(vaginal)*. Mientras se pone la bata, le vamos a sacar sangre para ver si está embarazada o tiene algún problema *(o tiene anemia, o hacerle un conteo de glóbulos rojos)*. También le vamos a hacer un ultrasonido del estómago. Es posible que usted esté embarazada. Si es así, tenemos que examinarla para estar seguros de que el bebé está en el lugar correcto. A veces el bebé puede estar en las trompas de Falopio en lugar del útero. El ultrasonido nos dirá dónde está el bebé. ¿Se puede poner esta bata, por favor? Volveré en unos minutos con una enfermera para hacer el examen.	Srta. Padilla, la vamos a examinar. Mientras se pone la bata, le vamos a sacar sangre para ver si está embarazada o tiene algún problema de salud. También le vamos a hacer un ultrasonido de la panza. Si está embarazada, tenemos que estar seguros de que el bebé está en el lugar correcto. A veces el bebé está en las trompas, en lugar de la matriz. El ultrasonido nos va a ayudar. Por favor, póngase la bata. Vuelvo en unos minutos con una enfermera para hacerle el examen.

PHYSICAL EXAM

You return accompanied by Ms. Carol Hoffman, LPN. Your patient is in a gown.

English	Spanish Formal	Spanish Informal
Q. Ms. Padilla. We are going to go ahead with the physical exam. This is Ms. Hoffman, the nurse who will be assisting me. We will first listen to your heart and lungs. Can you please sit on the table?	Srta. Padilla. Ahora vamos a hacer el examen físico. Esta es la Srta. Hoffman, la enfermera que me va a ayudar. Primero vamos a escuchar su corazón y sus pulmones. ¿Se puede sentar en la cama, por favor?	Ahora la vamos a examinar. Esta es la Srta. Hoffman, una enfermera que me va a ayudar. ¿Se puede sentar en la cama, por favor? Le voy a escuchar el corazón y los pulmones.
Q. Have you had a pelvic exam before?	¿Alguna vez le han hecho un examen de la pelvis?	¿Le han hecho un examen vaginal antes?
A. Yes. I had a PAP smear done about a year ago.	Sí, hace un año me hicieron un examen de Papanicolau.	Sí. Me hicieron el Pap el año pasado.
Q. Next we will do the pelvic exam. Can you please lie down on the table? Carol will help you.	Ahora le vamos a hacer el examen de la pelvis. ¿Se puede acostar en la cama, por favor? Carol le va a ayudar.	Ahora le vamos a hacer el examen vaginal. ¿Puede acostarse en la cama, por favor? Carol le va a ayudar.
Can you move your hips closer to the edge of the table?	¿Puede moverse para abajo, cerca del borde de la cama?	Muévase para abajo, hasta el borde de la cama.
(With the patient covered) Can you place your feet in the stirrups?	(Con la paciente cubierta) ¿Puede colocar los pies en los estribos?	¿Puede poner los pies sobre los estribos?
First we will do a bimanual exam where we use the gloved hand to do the pelvic exam while palpating the abdomen with the other hand. We can sometimes feel a mass this way and we can assess the size of the uterus, which may be enlarged if you are pregnant. Next we will place the speculum so we can look inside and see if there is any evidence of infection or pregnancy.	Primero le vamos a hacer un examen bi-manual; en una mano, me voy a poner un guante para examinar la vagina, y con la otra, le voy a palpar el abdomen. A veces podemos sentir una masa (bola) de esta manera y podemos evaluar el tamaño del útero, que puede estar agrandado si usted está embarazada. Después le vamos a colocar un espéculo para ver adentro y ver si hay evidencia de infección o embarazo.	Primero le vamos a hacer un examen con las dos manos; en una mano, me voy a poner un guante para examinar la vagina, y con la otra, le voy a tocar la panza. A veces se puede sentir si hay una bola. También se puede examinar el tamaño de la matriz, que puede estar grande si estuviera embarazada. Después le vamos a poner un espéculo para ver adentro y ver si está embarazada o tiene alguna infección.

FINDINGS

An ill-defined mass is present in the right lower quadrant on palpation. There is voluntary guarding present in the right lower quadrant without signs of peritonitis. Pelvic exam reveals no evidence of infection. Blood examination including pregnancy test and CBC is pending. The trans-vaginal ultrasound will be done in the next 15 minutes.

FOLLOW-UP

English	Spanish Formal	Spanish Informal
Explaining to the patient: We will have the results of the exams in the next 30 minutes. I am concerned about an ectopic	*Explicación a la paciente:* El resultado de los exámenes estará listo en treinta minutos. Yo estoy preocupado por la	*Con la paciente:* Los resultados de los exámenes estarán listos en media hora. Estoy preocupado porque puede ser un

English	Spanish Formal	Spanish Informal Continued
pregnancy, in other words, a pregnancy in the tube instead of in the uterus. The tube is very small so as the fetus grows the tube can stretch, causing pain and rupture. I called the obstetrician on call to see you. If it is an ectopic pregnancy, an operation is necessary because you can bleed if it ruptures.	posibilidad de que sea un embarazo ectópico, en otras palabras, un embarazo en la trompa de Falopio en vez de la matriz (útero). La trompa es muy pequeña, así que conforme el feto crece, la trompa se va estirando, causando dolor y ruptura. Llamé al médico obstetra que está de guardia para que la examine. Si es un embarazo ectópico, va a ser necesario hacer una operación porque usted puede sangrar si se rompe.	embarazo ectópico, o sea un embarazo en las trompas en lugar de dentro de la matriz. La trompa es muy pequeña y conforme el bebé va creciendo, la trompa se estira y se puede romper. Llamé al médico obstetra para que la examine. Si es un embarazo ectópico, le va a hacer una operación porque se puede romper y usted puede sangrar.
The other possibility is a twisted ovary or a ruptured cyst in the ovary. This can often be diagnosed by the ultrasound.	Las otras posibilidades son una torsión de ovario o la ruptura de un quiste de ovario. Esto se puede diagnosticar frecuentemente con un ultrasonido.	Otras posibilidades es que sea una torcedura del ovario o una ruptura de un quiste de ovario. Esto se puede diagnosticar con un ultrasonido.
An infection is unlikely due to the absence of fever and vaginal discharge. The ultrasound will help greatly in ruling out either one of the above possible diagnoses.	No creo que sea una infección porque usted no tiene fiebre ni secreción vaginal. El ultrasonido nos va a ayudar muchísimo para descartar cualquiera de estos posibles diagnósticos.	No pienso que sea una infección porque no tiene desecho por la vagina. El ultrasonido nos puede ayudar mucho para saber lo que es.

It is important to remember that in any woman of childbearing age who presents to the emergency room with abdominal pain, ectopic pregnancy is the number one diagnosis to rule out. Why? Because if it ruptures, the woman can die of exsanguination. In this case, the patient is stable hemodynamically. Her pulse and blood pressure are normal. If this same patient presented hypotensive and tachycardic, both signs of hypovolemia due to hemorrhage, then she would be taken immediately to the operating room without any diagnostic testing. The presumed diagnosis would be ruptured ectopic pregnancy. Any patient who presents with intra-abdominal bleeding needs to go to the operating room immediately. Minutes can often be the difference between life and death.

Symptoms of ectopic pregnancy include unilateral lower abdominal pain, vaginal spotting or cessation of the menstrual period, nausea, breast enlargement and tenderness as seen in normal pregnancy; hypotension, shock, and shoulder pain (due to blood irritating the diaphragm) may be present if the fallopian tube ruptures. However, the symptoms may be quite vague and non-specific, thus the clinician must maintain a high index of suspicion.

The number one risk factor for having a tubal pregnancy is a history of salpingitis, commonly termed pelvic inflammatory disease (PID). This is an infection usually sexually transmitted causing infection in the fallopian tube. The resultant scarring inhibits movement of the ovary, so fertilization occurs in the tube. Any pelvic scarring such as a history of appendicitis can cause the fallopian tube to kink, causing the same effect. The morning after pill and birth control pills containing progesterone also increase the risk of tubal pregnancy, if pregnancy does occur, due to the slowed movement of the ovum down the tube, resulting in an extra-uterine pregnancy.

If one suspects an ectopic pregnancy, a serum pregnancy test (β-HCG) should be ordered immediately. This is much more sensitive than urine β-HCG. A positive β-HCG tells you there is a pregnancy, but doesn't tell you if the pregnancy is in the tube or the uterus. Your physical exam in this case points to a tubal pregnancy due to the palpation of an adnexal (tubal) mass in the lower

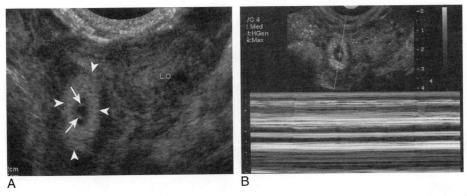

Figure 4-2. Unruptured tubal pregnancy in a 26-year-old nulliparous woman. **A,** Axial image of transvaginal US shows echogenic rim (*arrowheads*) and inner ring-shaped echo (*arrows*) suggesting extrauterine gestational sac and yolk sac, respectively. LO, left ovary. **B,** M-mode US demonstrates no cardiac activity within the small-sized echogenic lesion, suggesting a dead embryo in the extrauterine gestational sac. (From Kim SH, McClennan BL, Outwater EK: *Radiology Illustrated: Gynecologic Imaging.* Philadelphia, WB Saunders, 2005.)

abdomen. However, in almost 50% of patients, a mass cannot be palpated in a woman with an ectopic pregnancy. Thus, trans-vaginal ultrasonography is the mode of choice for imaging. If an intra-uterine pregnancy is seen, then the diagnosis of ectopic pregnancy is ruled out. If an intra-uterine pregnancy is not seen or a tubal pregnancy is visualized, then the diagnosis of tubal pregnancy is confirmed (Fig. 4-2).

The next step is consultation with the obstetric-gynecology consult on call. Although asymptomatic cases of tubal pregnancy have been treated non-operatively with methotrexate, the more accepted treatment, especially in the case of symptomatic tubal pregnancy, is surgery to remove the products of conception.

CASE 2: ENDOMETRIAL CANCER

CHIEF COMPLAINT

A 58-year-old female presents with vaginal bleeding. Her vital signs are normal.

HISTORY OF PRESENT ILLNESS

	English	Spanish Formal	Spanish Informal
Q.	Hello, Ms. Gomez, I am Dr. Adams. What brings you in to see us today?	Hola, Sra. Gómez, soy el Dr. Adams. ¿Por qué vino a vernos hoy?	Hola, Sra. Gómez, soy el Dr. Adams. ¿Por qué vino hoy?
A.	I started having vaginal bleeding two months ago.	Comencé a tener sangrados vaginales hace dos meses.	Desde hace dos meses, estoy sangrando por la vagina.
Q.	How old are you?	¿Qué edad tiene?	¿Cuántos años tiene?
A.	I am 58 years of age.	Tengo cincuenta y ocho años de edad.	Cincuenta y ocho años.
Q.	Are you still on your periods or have you passed through menopause?	¿Todavía le viene la menstruación o ya pasó por la menopausia?	¿Todavía le viene la regla o ya tuvo la menopausia?
A.	About four years ago my periods stopped when I went through menopause. That is	Hace cuatro años que dejé de tener la menstruación, cuando pasé por la	Desde hace cuatro años no me viene la regla. Por eso me preocupé cuando comencé a sangrar otra vez.

English	Spanish Formal	Spanish Informal	Continued
why I was so worried when the bleeding started again.	menopausia. Por eso es que estaba tan preocupada cuando comencé a sangrar otra vez.		
Q. Is it every day or is it intermittent?	¿Es todos los días o es intermitente?	¿Es todos los días o le viene y se le va?	
A. It is almost every day.	Es casi todos los días.	Casi todos los días.	
Q. Is it heavy bleeding or light, for instance "spotting."	¿Es un sangrado abundante o leve, como un "manchado"?	¿Sangra mucho o es sólo un "manchado"?	
A. It is more like spotting. It is not very heavy.	Es más como un manchado. No es muy abundante *(no es mucha cantidad)*.	No es mucho, es un "manchado."	
Q. Does anything make it worse, such as sexual intercourse?	¿Hay algo que lo hace peor, como cuando tiene relaciones sexuales?	¿Hay algo que lo empeora? ¿Sangra más cuando tiene relaciones sexuales?	
A. The bleeding is not related to intercourse.	El sangrado no está asociado a las relaciones sexuales.	No.	
Q. Have you been pregnant before and do you have children from these pregnancies?	¿Ha estado embarazada antes? ¿Tiene niños de estos embarazos?	¿Ha estado embarazada? ¿Tiene niños?	
A. Yes, three times, and all three children were born healthy.	Sí, tres veces, y todos los niños nacieron saludables.	Sí, tres veces. Tengo tres hijos y nacieron normales.	
Q. Do you take estrogens?	¿Está tomando estrógenos?	¿Toma estrógenos, hormonas?	
A. I take estrogens that were given to me for hot flashes of menopause four years ago. I also take one aspirin a day for my heart.	Tomo estrógenos que me recetaron para "los calores" de la menopausia hace cuatro años. También tomo una aspirina diaria para el corazón.	Tomo estrógenos desde hace cuatro años para "los calores". También tomo aspirina para el corazón.	
Q. Is the bleeding getting better or worse?	¿El sangrado está mejorando o empeorando?	¿El sangrado está mejor o peor?	
A. It is a little worse now than when it started.	Es un poco peor ahora que cuando comenzó.	Es peor ahora que cuando empezó.	
Q. Have you ever had abnormal vaginal bleeding before, including heavy periods prior to menopause?	¿Alguna vez ha tenido sangrados vaginales anormales, incluyendo menstruaciones abundantes, antes de la menopausia?	¿Alguna vez tuvo sangrados anormales antes de la menopausia, incluyendo reglas abundantes?	
A. I had heavy periods when I was younger but these completely stopped after I went through menopause.	Tuve reglas abundantes cuando era más joven, pero dejaron de venir completamente después de la menopausia.	Tuve reglas "fuertes" cuando era más joven, pero dejaron de venir después de la menopausia.	
Q. About how old were you when you had your first period and what age were you when they stopped?	¿Qué edad tenía cuando tuvo la primera menstruación y a que edad le dejaron de venir?	¿Cuántos años tenía cuando tuvo la primera regla y a qué edad le dejaron de venir?	
A. I was about 14 years old when I had my first period and they stopped when I was 54 years old.	Tenía catorce años cuando tuve la primera menstruación y me dejaron de venir cuando tenía cincuenta y cuatro años.	La primera regla me vino a los catorce años. La regla me dejó de venir a los cincuenta y cuatro.	
Q. Have you ever had any gynecologic diseases such as ovarian, cervical or vaginal cancer?	¿Alguna vez ha tenido una enfermedad ginecológica, como cáncer del cerviz, el ovario o la vagina?	¿Alguna vez ha tenido una enfermedad del aparato reproductivo, como cáncer del cuello de la matriz, la vagina o los ovarios?	
A. No, I have never been diagnosed with cancer.	No, nunca me han diagnosticado cáncer.	No, nunca he tenido cáncer.	

	English	Spanish Formal	Spanish Informal
Q.	Do you have a PAP smear done on a yearly basis?	¿Le hacen un examen de Papanicolau todos los años?	¿Se hace examen de Papanicolau todos los años?
A.	Yes. The last PAP smear I had was two years ago and it was normal.	Sí. El último Papanicolau que tuve fue hace dos años y era normal.	Hace dos años me hicieron el último Papanicolau y fue normal.
Q.	Is there any associated abdominal pain or bloating with the bleeding?	¿Tiene dolor abdominal o siente el estómago inflamado cuando está sangrando?	¿Tiene dolor de panza o se siente "empanzada" cuando está sangrando?
A.	No, I have had no stomach pains.	No, nunca he tenido dolores de estómago.	No.
Q.	Do you have any symptoms of fatigue, weakness, tiredness, or light-headedness?	¿Tiene síntomas de fatiga, debilidad, cansancio o mareo?	¿Se siente cansada, débil o mareada?
A.	I feel tired all the time. I sleep a lot more than before. I feel like I have no energy.	Me siento cansada todo el tiempo. Duermo mucho más que antes. Siento como que no tuviera energía.	Me siento cansada todo el tiempo. Me ha dado mucho sueño y me siento muy débil.
Q.	Have you noticed excessive bleeding or bruising in the past few months?	¿Ha notado sangrado excesivo o magulladuras (moretones) en los últimos meses?	¿Ha notado moretones en la piel o mucho sangrado en los últimos días?
A.	No, I haven't noted any change.	No, no he notado ningún cambio.	No.
Q.	Have you noticed any rectal bleeding?	¿Ha notado sangrado por el recto?	¿Ha sangrado por el recto?
A.	I have not noted any rectal bleeding.	No he notado ningún sangrado por el recto.	No, no he sangrado por el recto.
Q.	Have you had a colonoscopy in the last five years?	¿Le han hecho una colonoscopía en los últimos cinco años?	¿Alguna vez le han hecho una colonoscopía?
A.	I had a colonoscopy three years ago and it was normal.	Me hicieron una colonoscopía hace tres años y era normal.	Me hicieron una colonoscopía hace tres años y fue normal.
Q.	Do you have any medical problems such as diabetes, thyroid disease, or liver disease?	¿Tiene alguna otra enfermedad, como diabetes, enfermedad de la tiroides o del hígado?	¿Padece de alguna otra enfermedad, como diabetes, de la tiroides o del hígado?
A.	I was told my sugar was high but it has been controlled by diet. My sugars have been normal on my last checkups.	Me dijeron que tenía el azúcar alto, pero se ha controlado con la dieta. Las últimas veces que me han examinado el azúcar ha estado normal.	Me dijeron que tenía el azúcar alto, pero estaba controlándolo con la dieta. En los últimos exámenes he tenido el azúcar normal.
Q.	Do you have any other medical problems such as heart, lung or abdominal disease?	¿Tiene algún otro problema de salud, como una enfermedad del corazón, los pulmones o el abdomen?	¿Padece de alguna otra enfermedad, como del corazón, los pulmones o la panza?
A.	I have high blood pressure controlled by diet.	Tengo la presión alta y me controlo con la dieta.	Tengo presión alta. Me la controlo con la dieta.
Q.	Have you lost any weight due to a loss of appetite?	¿Ha perdido peso por falta de apetito?	¿Ha perdido peso por falta de apetito?
A.	My weight is about the same but I have lost my appetite somewhat.	Mi peso es casi el mismo, pero he perdido un poco el apetito.	Peso casi igual, pero no me dan ganas de comer.
Q.	Do you smoke or drink alcohol?	¿Toma licor o fuma cigarrillos?	¿Toma o fuma?
A.	I stopped smoking 12 years ago and drink very rarely.	Dejé de fumar hace doce años y tomo licor muy de vez en cuando.	Dejé el cigarrillo hace doce años. Tomo muy de vez en cuando.
Q.	Ms. Gomez, I am going to return with Carol our nurse to perform a physical exam. Can you please change into the gown, and I will be right back.	Sra. Gómez, voy a regresar para hacerle un examen físico. ¿Puede ponerse esta bata, por favor?, que yo regreso en un momento.	Regresaré en un momento para hacerle un examen. Póngase esta bata, por favor.

RESULTS OF THE PHYSICAL EXAM

There is a little blood in the vaginal canal. Otherwise, the exam is normal. There are no palpable adnexal masses on bimanual palpation. Rectal exam is likewise normal, with no evidence of blood in the stool. The vaginal lining and cervix appear normal.

DIFFERENTIAL DIAGNOSIS

- Endometrial cancer
- Fibroids (leiomyoma of the uterus)
- Endometrial hyperplasia
- Endometrial polyps
- Cervical-vaginal etiology

Abnormal vaginal bleeding in the young, pre-menopausal woman is most commonly a benign condition (most commonly dysfunctional uterine bleeding due to anovulation). In this situation, the corpus luteum fails to form, resulting in failure of progesterone secretion. The unopposed estradiol causes hyperplasia of the endometrium. As noted above, in the young woman, more serious conditions such as ectopic pregnancy need to be ruled out.

However, in the postmenopausal woman, like our patient above, vaginal bleeding is cancer until proven otherwise. The most common cancer in this setting is endometrial, the cells of which line the uterus. Endometrial cancer is the fourth most common cancer in women preceded by breast, pulmonary, and colorectal. Risk factors center around increased exposure to estrogen unopposed by progesterone. Thus, questions will center around this risk factor, such as whether your patient takes estrogens and onset of menses and menopause (increased exposure to estrogen with early menses and late menopause). Nulliparous woman have increased exposure to estrogen versus women who have had multiple births. During pregnancy, progesterone levels rise in relation to estrogen, conferring a protective effect on the endometrial lining. Diabetes and obesity increase the risk of endometrial cancer. Both conditions are associated with a higher level of estrogens. Prior to the development of endometrial cancer, the endometrial lining goes through the stages of hyperplasia prior to becoming malignant. About 10% of cancers arise de novo in normal tissue. It is important to note that only 10% to 20% of patients with vaginal bleeding in the postmenopausal state will have malignancy. Other conditions such as leiomyoma (fibroids), endometrial hyperplasia and polyps, and inflammation of the vaginal mucosa can present with these symptoms. In addition, 10% of women with endometrial carcinoma will present with purulent, pink-tinged drainage. In summary, the take-home message in the postmenopausal woman who presents with bleeding: Rule Out Cancer. This certainly can be done on an outpatient basis.

FOLLOW-UP

English	Spanish Formal	Spanish Informal
To the patient: I am concerned about the abnormal vaginal bleeding that you are having. This may indicate something benign	*A la paciente:* Estoy preocupado por el sangrado vaginal anormal que usted ha tenido. Esto puede indicar algo benigno,	*A la paciente:* Me tiene preocupado el sangrado vaginal que tiene usted. Puede ser algo benigno, como una irritación, o

English	Spanish Formal	Spanish Informal
such as irritation or a benign growth such as a polyp in the uterus. On my exam, the vagina and cervix appeared normal. The bleeding may be due to a cancer in the uterus. I didn't see any abnormality in the vagina or cervix, so it is most likely from the uterus.	como una irritación, o un crecimiento benigno, como un pólipo en el útero. En el examen, la vagina y el cerviz parecen normales. El sangrado puede ser debido a un cáncer del útero. No observé ninguna anormalidad en la vagina o el cerviz, así que lo más posible es que sea del útero.	un pólipo de la matriz. Durante el examen que le hice, la vagina y el cerviz parecen normales. El sangrado puede ser por un cáncer de la matriz. No observé nada anormal en la vagina o el cuello, así que posiblemente es de la matriz.
Your fatigue may be due to the chronic or slow loss of blood. We will go ahead and draw some blood to check your blood count and to see if your blood is clotting normally. Also, due to the fatigue, we will do a blood test to check your thyroid function. I will schedule you for an ultrasound of the lower abdomen, which will allow us to see the uterus, tubes, and ovaries. We did a PAP smear during the pelvic exam and these results should be available.	La fatiga se puede deber a la pérdida crónica o lenta de sangre. Vamos a sacarle sangre para hacer unas pruebas y examinar su conteo de glóbulos rojos y ver si su sangre coagula normalmente. También, debido al cansancio, vamos a hacerle un examen de sangre para examinar la función de la glándula tiroides. Voy a hacerle una cita para un ultrasonido del abdomen inferior, que nos permitirá ver el útero, los tubos y los ovarios. Le hicimos una prueba de Papanicolau durante el examen de la pelvis y los resultados deberían estar listos.	El cansancio posiblemente sea por la pérdida crónica de sangre. Vamos a hacerle unos exámenes de sangre para ver si tiene anemia, problemas de coagulación y de la tiroides. También le voy a hacer una cita para un ultrasonido de la panza. Nos va a ayudar a ver cómo están la matriz, los tubos y los ovarios. Le hicimos un Papanicolau durante el examen y los resultados deberían estar listos.
I will make a referral to see Dr. Poden, a gynecologist who specializes in this area. They will most likely do an ultrasound of the inside of the uterus and possibly take some biopsies of the lining of the uterus. They do these procedures in the office in most cases and you may even have the answer as to what is causing the bleeding the day you see the gynecologist. As I said before, often the cause of vaginal bleeding is benign, not due to cancer, and the treatment may be very simple; however, it is important to make sure it is not a more serious cause such as cancer. Do you have any questions?	Voy a hacer una referencia para ver al Dr. Poden, un ginecólogo que se especializa en esa área. Lo más probable es que ellos le hagan un ultrasonido de la parte de adentro del útero y posiblemente tomarán muestras para biopsias de la superficie del útero. Ellos realizan este procedimiento en el consultorio la mayoría de las veces y es posible que hasta le puedan contestar qué es lo que está causando el sangrado el mismo día que usted vea al ginecólogo. Como dije antes, con frecuencia la causa del sangrado vaginal es benigna, no es por cáncer, y el tratamiento puede ser muy sencillo; sin embargo, es importante que esté segura de que no es algo más serio, como un cáncer. ¿Tiene alguna pregunta?	La voy a mandar para que la vea el Dr. Poden, un ginecólogo especialista. Posiblemente le va a hacer un ultrasonido de la matriz y le tomará muestras para una biopsia. Por lo general, ellos hacen este estudio en el consultorio, así que es posible que le pueda decir cuál es la causa del sangrado el mismo día. Como dije antes, por lo general la causa del sangrado vaginal es benigna y no se debe a un cáncer. El tratamiento puede ser muy sencillo. Sin embargo, es muy importante que estemos seguros de que no es un problema más serio, como un cáncer. ¿Tiene preguntas?
Q. If it is cancer, what is the treatment?	Si es cáncer, ¿cuál es el tratamiento?	De ser cáncer, ¿cuáles el tratamiento?
A. I am not a specialist in this area, but I believe it would depend on the stage of the cancer or how advanced it is. Dr. Poden will certainly go over all the options if this turns out to be the case, but again, many of the causes of this type of bleeding are benign.	Yo no soy especialista en esta área, pero creo que todo depende del estadio del cáncer o qué tan avanzado esté. Ciertamente, el Dr. Poden le explicará todas las opciones, si este fuera el caso. Pero, otra vez, muchas veces la causa de este tipo de sangrado es benigna.	No soy especialista en ginecología, pero creo que todo depende de la etapa de desarrollo del cáncer o qué tan avanzado esté. Si fuera necesario, el Dr. Poden le explicará todas las opciones. Pero, como le dije antes, muchas veces la causa de este tipo de sangrado es benigna.

CASE 3: PELVIC INFLAMMATORY DISEASE

CHIEF COMPLAINT

Sylvia Robles, an 18-year-old female patient, presents to your office with a chief complaint of fever, lower abdominal pain bilaterally, and vaginal discharge. She is accompanied by her parents.

HISTORY

English	Spanish Formal	Spanish Informal
Q. Hello (to all three). I am Dr. Roberts. (To Sylvia) What brings you to see us today, Ms. Robles?	Hola (a los tres), soy el Dr. Roberts. (Dirigiéndose a Sylvia) ¿Por qué viene a vernos hoy, Srta. Robles?	Hola, soy el Dr. Roberts. Srta. Robles, ¿por qué viene a vernos hoy?
A. I have had fever and chills and abdominal pain for the past three days. The pain has been getting worse. I have also had a discharge.	He tenido fiebre, escalofríos y dolor en el abdomen los últimos tres días. El dolor ha empeorado. También he tenido flujo.	He tenido calentura, "calofríos" y dolor de panza desde hace tres días. El dolor se ha hecho peor. También tengo desecho.
Q. How old are you?	¿Qué edad tiene?	¿Cuántos años tiene?
A. I am 18 years old.	Tengo dieciocho años de edad.	Dieciocho años.
Q. Where is the discharge coming from?	¿De dónde viene el flujo?	¿De dónde es el desecho?
A. The discharge is from the vagina.	El flujo es de la vagina.	De la vagina.
Q. Does it have a bad odor?	¿Tiene mal olor?	¿Huele mal?
A. Yes, very bad especially in the last day.	Sí, huele muy mal, especialmente desde ayer.	Sí, es peor desde ayer.
Q. What color is it?	¿De qué color es?	¿De qué color?
A. Yellowish-white.	Es amarrillo con blanco.	Amarillo con blanco.
Q. When was your last period and was it normal?	¿Cuándo fue su última menstruación? ¿Le vino normal?	¿Cuándo tuvo la última regla? ¿Fue normal?
A. My last period was about two weeks ago and it was normal.	Mi última menstruación fue hace dos semanas y fue normal.	Hace dos semanas tuve la última regla. Me vino normal.
Q. Have you had any bleeding from the vagina since then?	¿Ha tenido algún sangrado por la vagina desde entonces?	Después de la regla, ¿ha tenido sangrado por la vagina?
A. No, I have had no bleeding.	No, no he tenido ningún sangrado.	No.
Q. (To the parents): There are certain very personal questions I have to ask in order to arrive at the right diagnosis and give your daughter the best treatment I can. (To Sylvia): Are you more comfortable with your parents here?	(A los padres): Hay varias preguntas muy personales que tengo que hacer para llegar al diagnóstico correcto y darle a su hija el mejor tratamiento que le puedo ofrecer. (A Sylvia): ¿Se siente más cómoda con sus padres aquí?	(A los padres): Tengo que hacerle unas preguntas personales a Sylvia para saber lo que tiene y darle el tratamiento correcto. (A Sylvia): Sylvia, ¿se siente más cómoda si sus padres se quedan en el consultorio?
A. Yes, I would like them to be here.	Sí, quiero que se queden conmigo.	Sí, quiero que se queden.
Q. Have you ever been pregnant before?	¿Alguna vez ha estado embarazada?	¿Ha estado embarazada?
A. No, I have never been pregnant.	No, nunca he estado embarazada.	No.
Q. Is there a chance you might be pregnant?	¿Hay alguna posibilidad de que pudiera estar embarazada?	¿Hay algún "chance" de que usted pueda estar embarazada?
A. No, there is no chance.	No, ninguna posibilidad.	No.
Q. Have you had sexual relations in the past and, if so, how long ago was the last time?	¿Ha tenido relaciones sexuales en el pasado? Y de ser así, ¿cuándo fue la última vez?	¿Ha tenido relaciones sexuales? ¿Cuándo fue la última vez?
A. About 2 weeks ago was the last time.	La última vez fue hace dos semanas.	Sí, hace dos semanas fue la última vez.

English	Spanish Formal	Spanish Informal
Q. Do you use some form of contraception?	¿Usa algún método anticonceptivo?	¿Usa algo para evitar el embarazo?
A. I take birth control pills.	Tomo pastillas anticonceptivas.	Tomo pastillas.
Q. Do you use condoms during sex?	¿Usa condones cuando tiene relaciones sexuales?	¿Usa condones?
A. Sometimes we use condoms, sometimes we don't.	A veces usamos condones y a veces, no.	De vez en cuando.
Q. Have you had more than one sexual partner in the past month?	¿Ha tenido más de un compañero sexual en el último mes?	¿Ha tenido relaciones con más de una persona en el último mes?
A. No, I have a boyfriend and we have been together for the past year.	No, yo tengo novio y tenemos un año de estar juntos.	No, sólo con mi novio. Tenemos un año de estar juntos.
Q. Have you ever had a vaginal infection before or any type of gynecologic problems?	¿Alguna vez ha tenido una infección vaginal o algún otro tipo de problema ginecológico?	¿Alguna vez ha tenido una infección por la vagina u otro problema ginecológico?
A. I had a yeast infection a year ago after I took antibiotics for bronchitis.	Tuve una candidiasis vaginal hace un año después de tomar un tratamiento de antibióticos.	Tuve un hongo hace un año porque tuve que tomar un tratamiento de antibióticos.
Q. You mentioned you have had abdominal pain for the past three days and it's gotten worse. Where did it start and where is it located now?	Usted dijo que había tenido dolor abdominal los últimos tres días y que había empeorado. ¿Dónde le comenzó y dónde está localizado ahora?	¿Dónde le comenzó el dolor de panza y dónde lo siente ahora?
A. It started all over the lower part of my stomach and it is still located in the same place but it's a lot worse.	Me comenzó por toda la parte de abajo del estómago y todavía está en el mismo lugar, pero es peor.	Me empezó en la parte de abajo de la panza y todavía esta ahí, pero ahora es peor.
Q. What makes it better or worse?	¿Qué lo mejora? ¿Qué lo empeora?	¿Qué lo hace mejor y qué lo hace peor?
A. It is better when I lie still and hurts when I move around.	Es mejor cuando me acuesto quieta *(sin moverme)* y duele cuando me muevo.	Me duele más cuando me muevo y se me alivia un poco cuando estoy quieta *(quedita).*
Q. Are there any other associated symptoms such as nausea, vomiting, or diarrhea?	¿Tiene algún otro síntoma, como náusea, vómito o diarrea?	¿Tiene otros síntomas, como ganas de vomitar o diarrea?
A. I have had some nausea today and vomited once. I have no diarrhea.	He tenido algo de náusea hoy y vomité una vez. No he tenido diarrea.	Hoy tengo ganas de vomitar y me vomité una vez. No tengo diarrea.
Q. Have you had any problems urinating such as burning on urination, urinating more often than before, or cloudiness of the urine?	¿Ha tenido algún problema para orinar, como ardor al orinar, orinar con más frecuencia que antes u orina turbia?	¿Ha tenido algún problema al orinar, como quemazón, orinar con más frecuencia u orina turbia?
A. I have had no problem with urination.	No he tenido ningún problema de orina.	No.
Q. Have you ever had surgery before?	¿Ha tenido alguna cirugía antes?	¿Alguna vez la han operado?
A. I had a tonsillectomy when I was five years old.	Tuve una amigdalectomía cuando tenía cinco años.	Me sacaron las glándulas cuando tenía cinco años.
Q. Do you have any medical problems such as lung or heart disease, diabetes?	¿Tiene alguna enfermedad de los pulmones, el corazón o la diabetes?	¿Padece de los pulmones, el corazón o la diabetes?
A. Not now. I had asthma as a child but haven't had any problems for around the past 10 years.	Ahora no. Tuve asma cuando era niña, pero no he tenido problemas desde hace como diez años.	No. Tuve asma, pero no he tenido problemas en los últimos diez años.

	English	Spanish Formal	Spanish Informal Continued
Q.	Do you have any allergies to medication?	¿Es alérgica a algún medicamento?	¿Es alérgica a alguna medicina?
A.	No, not that I know of.	No que yo sepa.	No.
Q.	We will do a physical exam, including a pelvic exam. Can you change into a gown please? And I will return with Carol, one of the nurses who works here in the clinic.	Vamos a hacerle un examen físico, incluyendo un examen pélvico. ¿Se puede poner una bata, por favor? Y yo regresaré con Carol, una de las enfermeras que trabaja en la clínica.	Le voy a hacer un examen vaginal. ¿Se puede poner esta bata, por favor? Yo regresaré en un momento con Carol, una enfermera de la clínica.
	(To the parents): If you can wait in the waiting room until after the exam, I will come and get you and bring you back to the room.	(A los padres): Si pueden esperar en la sala de espera hasta después del examen, yo los vendré a buscar para que vengan de nuevo al consultorio.	(A los padres): Señores padres, ¿pueden quedarse en la sala de espera hasta que termine? Yo los voy a venir a buscar para que regresen al consultorio.

PHYSICAL EXAM RESULTS

Vital signs: Temp. 38.9°C, P 94, BP 110/64, R 22. Tenderness throughout the lower abdomen with involuntary guarding and rebound. Pelvic exam reveals bilateral adnexal tenderness and purulent vaginal discharge, as well as discharge coming from the cervical os (Fig. 4-3). There is severe pain on moving the cervix. A gram stain and culture of the vaginal secretions are sent.

This is the classic picture of salpingitis, more commonly called pelvic inflammatory disease (PID). It is typically transmitted sexually and begins initially as an infection in the vagina or cervix that ascends into the uterus and the fallopian tubes. Any condition that opens the cervical os such as occurs during the menstrual period increases the risk of this retrograde flow. In addition, changes in the vaginal-cervical flora as occurs with antibiotic therapy may cause overgrowth of certain bacteria causing salpingitis. While the vast majority of infections in the fallopian tube are sexually transmitted, it is estimated that 10% to 20% of PID is a non-sexually transmitted disease (STD). The two most common bacteria involved in PID include *Nisseria gonorrhea* and

Figure 4-3. Laparoscopy in a patient with pelvic inflammatory disease. (From Copeland L: *Textbook of Gynecology*, ed 2. Philadelphia, WB Saunders, 1999.)

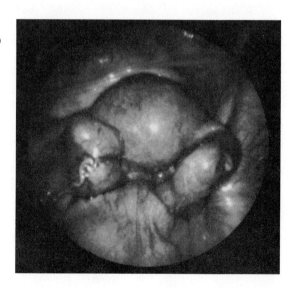

Chlamydia trachomatis, although other bacteria are often also involved, such as anerobic bacteria. Thus, these infections are usually polymicrobial.

Risk factors for salpingitis include young age (15 to 25), multiple sexual partners, and non-use of condoms. It is much less common in postmenopausal women and very rare during pregnancy, during which time the mucous of the cervix becomes thick, preventing ascent of infection.

The most common clinical finding in patients with PID is bilateral lower abdominal pain. In about 80% of patients, there will also be purulent discharge coming from the cervical os. Fever is often present. Nausea and vomiting, as noted in our patient, is a later presentation as the disease progresses and peritonitis occurs, causing an ileus. Often, symptoms will present at the end of the menstrual period, when progesterone levels are low, causing a change in the cervical mucous and predisposing the patient to ascent of infection from the vaginal-cervical canal.

On physical exam, bilateral lower abdominal tenderness is present. It can be severe as in the above patient, presenting with signs of peritonitis due to inflammation of the tubes and anterior abdominal wall, producing involuntary guarding, also termed rigidity. Pain on cervical motion is often severe and pus can often be seen coming from the cervical os.

It is very interesting that in about 10% to 15% of patients minimal symptomatology is noted.

DIFFERENTIAL DIAGNOSIS

In the differential diagnosis, one must rule out ectopic pregnancy, a life-threatening disease, although in our patient, the severe abdominal pain coupled with purulent vaginal discharge make PID more likely. It is important to note that both diseases, PID and ectopic pregnancy, may co-exist and make the diagnosis of ectopic pregnancy difficult if not considered. Appendicitis is also in the differential. The symptoms of PID and appendicitis may make it difficult to distinguish one disease from the other. In PID the fever is usually higher than in appendicitis. In addition, in PID the pain is usually much more severe and with movement of the cervix during the pelvic exam, the pain is made much worse. Urinary tract infection also may present with fever and lower abdominal pain; however, usually dysuria and frequency of urination are present.

Thus, one should always order a β-HCG to rule out pregnancy. A cervical culture as well as gram stain should be done for *N. gonorrhea* and *C. trachomatis.* The finding of polymorphonuclear leukocytes on wet mount or saline preparation slide is supportive of the diagnosis of PID. A urine gram stain and culture as well as urine analysis should be done to rule out the diagnosis of urinary tract infection.

Imaging studies such as ultrasound are helpful in ruling out a tubo-ovarian abscess (TOA) which may form in the fallopian tube. Computed tomography, or CT scan, is helpful in the case above to rule out a ruptured appendix. It also visualizes the fallopian tube and can diagnose a TOA.

If there is doubt, the gold standard for diagnosing PID is laparoscopy, where one can directly visualize the tubes as well as the ovary and appendix (Fig. 4-4). Most often, this procedure is done when one cannot exclude the diagnosis of appendicitis. If present, the appendix can be removed laparoscopically.

FOLLOW-UP

English	Spanish Formal	Spanish Informal
(With the patient alone): It appears that you have a vaginal infection. We have sent a gram stain that will be examined shortly and a culture that will take a couple of days to get back. We will have blood drawn to check if you are pregnant, as well as a blood test to look for infection. I will go ahead and order an ultrasound to see if there is an abscess in the tubes connecting the uterus and ovaries. Although other possibilities exist, most likely you have infection in the tubes. This is usually sexually transmitted but can occur non-sexually also. The usual treatment when fever and severe abdominal pain are present is admission to the hospital for intravenous antibiotics. It is also important your boyfriend gets seen and treated. It goes without saying that you are not protected from diseases such as HIV, hepatitis, and syphilis. Before we call your parents back to the room, I need to know if you wish me to talk to them regarding what we have discussed. It is totally up to you if you wish me to discuss what you and I have discussed.	(Sólo con la paciente): Parece que usted tuviera una infección vaginal. Enviamos una muestra que será examinada dentro de un rato y un cultivo que va a tomar un par de días para regresar. Vamos a sacarle sangre para ver si está embarazada y si tiene una infección. Voy a ordenar un ultrasonido para ver si hay un absceso en los tubos que conectan al útero y los ovarios. Aunque existen otras posibilidades, lo más posible es que tenga una infección en los tubos. Por lo general, estas infecciones son de transmisión sexual pero pueden presentarse sin contacto sexual. El tratamiento usual cuando hay fiebre y dolor abdominal severo es internamiento en el hospital para darle antibióticos intravenosos. También es importante que veamos a su novio para darle tratamiento. No hay necesidad de decir que usted no está protegida de enfermedades como VIH, hepatitis y sífilis. Antes de llamar a sus padres de regreso al consultorio, necesito saber si quiere que les cuente lo que le acabo de decir. Todo depende de usted si quiere que les cuente lo que acabamos de conversar.	(Sólo con la paciente): Señorita, parece que tuviera una infección vaginal. Enviamos una muestra que van a examinar dentro de un rato y un cultivo que va a venir en dos días. También le vamos a hacer un examen de sangre para ver si está embarazada o si tiene infección. Voy a pedir un ultrasonido para ver si hay un absceso en las trompas que conectan la matriz con los ovarios. Aunque hay otras posibilidades, creo que tiene una infección en los tubos. Por lo general, son de transmisión sexual, pero pueden ser por otra causa. Cuando hay fiebre y dolor de panza fuerte, ingresamos a la paciente para ponerle antibióticos por la vena. También es importante que veamos a su novio para darle tratamiento. No hay necesidad de decirle que usted no está protegida de enfermedades como el VIH, la hepatitis o la sífilis. Antes de hablar de nuevo con sus padres, quiero saber si usted quiere que yo les diga lo que acabamos de hablar. Todo depende de usted.
(Patient): Thank you. I would like to talk to them myself if that is okay.	Gracias. Me gustaría hablar con ellos yo misma, si está bien para usted.	Gracias, pero prefiero hablar con ellos yo misma.
Of course. We will go ahead and get the antibiotics started and give you something for the pain.	Por supuesto. Vamos a seguir adelante, comenzaremos con los antibióticos y le daremos algo para el dolor.	Está bien. Vamos a comenzar con los antibióticos y le vamos a dar algo para el dolor.

CASE 4: PREGNANCY

The final case involves the follow-up of a pregnant patient commonly seen in practice today, generally in the emergency room, due to the common event of a lack of medical insurance. Many people today get all their medical care in this setting, owing to the fact that the ER, by law, has to treat all patients regardless of financial circumstances.

CHIEF COMPLAINT

A 31-year-old woman presents to the clinic for follow-up of her pregnancy. This is her first visit.

HISTORY

	English	Spanish Formal	Spanish Informal
Q.	Hello, Ms. Ley, I am Dr. Jones.	Hola, Srta. Ley, soy el Doctor Jones.	Hola, Srta. Ley, soy el Dr. Jones.
A.	Hello, doctor.	Hola, doctor.	Hola, doctor.
Q.	How many weeks are you pregnant?	¿Cuántas semanas de embarazo tiene?	¿Cuánto tiene de embarazo?
A.	I am not sure, my last period was about six weeks ago.	No estoy segura, mi última menstruación fue hace seis semanas.	No sé. Tuve la última regla hace seis semanas.
Q.	How do you know you are pregnant?	¿Cómo sabe que está embarazada?	¿Está segura de que está embarazada?
A.	I bought a urine test at the pharmacy and it came out positive.	Compré una prueba de orina en la farmacia y me salió positiva.	Me hice una prueba de orina de farmacia y fue positiva.
Q.	Is this your first pregnancy?	¿Este es su primer embarazo?	¿Es su primer embarazo?
A.	No, I have one other child.	No, tengo otro niño.	No, tengo un hijo.
Q.	Have you ever had a miscarriage or spontaneous abortion?	¿Alguna vez ha tenido una pérdida o un aborto espontáneo?	¿Ha tenido pérdidas o abortos espontáneos?
A.	I had one miscarriage when I was 20 years old.	Tuve un aborto espontáneo cuando tenía veinte años.	Tuve una pérdida a los veinte años.
Q.	Did you have any problems with your prior pregnancy such as high blood pressure or elevated sugars?	¿Tuvo algún problema con los embarazos anteriores, como presión alta o azúcar elevado?	En los embarazos anteriores, ¿tuvo algún problema, como aumento del azúcar o la presión?
A.	No, I had no problems.	No, no tuve problemas.	No.
Q.	Was the baby full term or premature?	¿El bebé fue de término o prematuro?	¿El bebé nació de cuarenta semanas o se vino antes de tiempo?
A.	The baby was full term.	Fue de término.	De cuarenta semanas.
Q.	Did your baby have any problems at birth such as turning yellow or problems breathing?	¿Tuvo su bebé algún problema al nacer, como dificultad para respirar o ponerse amarillo?	¿Tuvo su bebé algún problema al nacer, como problemas para respirar o ponerse de color amarillo?
A.	He was fine after birth.	No tuvo problemas después de nacer.	No.
Q.	Are you doing well with the pregnancy? Have you had any nausea or vomiting?	¿Ha tenido algún problema durante el embarazo? ¿Ha tenido náuseas o vómito?	¿Cómo le va con el embarazo? ¿Ha tenido ganas de vomitar o vomitó?
A.	Yes. I am nauseated every morning and vomit at least once. By afternoon I feel a lot better.	Sí, me dan nauseas todas las mañanas y vomito por lo menos una vez. Me siento mejor por la tarde.	Sí, tengo ganas de vomitar por la mañana y vomito por lo menos una vez. Me siento mejor en la tarde.
Q.	Have you lost or gained weight over the past month?	¿Ha perdido o ganado peso el último mes?	¿Ha subido o bajado de peso?
A.	I have lost about five pounds. I feel so sick to my stomach it is hard to eat.	He perdido como cinco libras. Me siento tan enferma del estómago que me cuesta comer.	He perdido cinco libras. Me dan tantas ganas de vomitar que me cuesta comer.

	English	Spanish Formal	Spanish Informal	Continued
Q.	Have you noted swelling in your breasts and discomfort?	¿Ha notado molestias o inflamación en los senos?	¿Ha tenido molestias o hinchazón del busto?	
A.	Yes, especially over the last week.	Sí, especialmente en la última semana.	Sí, más esta semana.	
Q.	Have you noted any vaginal bleeding, "spotting," or discharge recently?	¿Ha notado sangrado, "manchado" o flujo por la vagina recientemente?	¿Ha tenido sangrado, "manchado" o desecho por la vagina últimamente?	
A.	No, I have had no vaginal discharge.	No, no he tenido flujo vaginal.	No.	
Q.	Have you had any abdominal pain or cramping?	¿Ha tenido dolor de estómago (abdominal) o cólicos?	¿Ha tenido dolor de vientre o retortijones?	
A.	No, I have not noticed any pains in my stomach.	No, no he tenido ningún dolor de estómago.	Tampoco.	
Q.	Prior to your pregnancy were you using any form of birth control such as condoms or birth control pills?	¿Antes del embarazo estaba usando algún método anticonceptivo, como condones o pastillas anticonceptivas?	¿Antes del embarazo estaba usando algún método para evitar el embarazo, como pastillas o condones?	
A.	I was using the pill but I must have forgotten to take it.	Estaba usando pastillas anticonceptivas, pero se me deben de haber olvidado.	Estaba tomando pastillas, pero seguro se me olvidaron.	
Q.	Do you have one partner or more than one?	¿Usted tiene sólo una pareja o más de una?	¿Usted tiene sólo un compañero o más de uno?	
A.	I have a boyfriend but I have had one other partner during this time.	Tengo un novio, pero también he tenido otra pareja en este tiempo.	Tengo un novio. También he tenido otro compañero últimamente.	
Q.	Do you have any medical problems such as diabetes, high blood pressure, heart or lung disease?	¿Tiene algún problema de salud, como diabetes, presión alta o alguna enfermedad del corazón o los pulmones?	¿Padece de diabetes, presión alta, del corazón o de los pulmones?	
A.	No, I am in good health.	No, tengo buena salud.	No.	
Q.	Have you ever had surgery?	¿Ha tenido alguna cirugía?	¿Alguna vez la han operado?	
A.	I had tubes put in my ears when I was three. I had my appendix taken out when I was 10 years old for appendicitis.	Me pusieron tubos en los oídos cuando tenía tres años. Me sacaron el apéndice cuando tenía diez años por una apendicitis.	A los tres años me pusieron tubos en los oídos. Me operaron del apéndice cuando tenía diez años por una apendicitis.	
Q.	Was the appendix ruptured?	¿Tuvo ruptura del apéndice?	¿Se le rompió el apéndice?	
A.	No, I don't think so.	No, yo no creo.	No.	
Q.	Do you smoke or drink alcohol?	¿Fuma cigarrillos o toma alcohol?	¿Fuma o toma licor?	
A.	I drink occasionally but have stopped since I realized I was pregnant.	Tomo de vez en cuando, pero lo dejé desde que me di cuenta de que estaba embarazada.	A veces tomo licor, pero lo dejé desde que me dijeron que estaba embarazada.	
Q.	Do you take any medications?	¿Toma algún medicamento?	¿Toma alguna medicina?	
A.	No, just a multivitamin.	No, sólo multi-vitaminas.	Sólo multi-vitaminas.	
Q.	Is there any history of birth diseases such as Down syndrome in your family?	¿Alguien en su familia ha tenido problemas congénitos, como síndrome de Down?	¿Alguien en su familia ha tenido problemas del nacimiento, como síndrome de Down?	
A.	I have a cousin on my mother's side with Down syndrome.	Tengo un primo de la familia de mi mamá que padece de síndrome de Down.	Tengo un primo de parte de mi mamá que tiene síndrome de Down.	
Q.	Ms. Ley, I am going to go ahead and do a physical exam including a pelvic exam to see how the pregnancy is doing. I will be back with Carol Hoffman, the nurse who works in the clinic. Can you change into a gown please?	Srta. Ley, le voy a hacer un examen físico, incluyendo un examen pélvico (vaginal) para ver cómo va el embarazo. Regresaré con Carol Hoffman, la enfermera que trabaja en la clínica. ¿Se puede poner esta bata, por favor?	Srta. Ley, le voy a hacer un examen para ver cómo va el embarazo. Regresaré con Carol Hoffman, la enfermera. ¿Se puede poner esta bata, por favor?	

PHYSICAL EXAM

After examining the heart, lungs and the abdomen, a pelvic exam is done. The findings on the pelvic exam are non-specific. The cervical os is closed; no blood or discharge is noted. The uterus is normal size.

FOLLOW-UP

English	Spanish Formal	Spanish Informal
Ms. Ley, we will check your serum to confirm the diagnosis of pregnancy. In addition, we will draw blood to check your hemoglobin and hematocrit. Sometimes these levels can be low if you lose a lot of blood during your period. It is also important to check your glucose or sugar level. We will also check your urine to make sure there is no protein or sugar in the urine. We will do an ultrasound in four weeks. I would like to see you back in a month. If you develop any problems sooner such as vaginal bleeding or discharge, cramping abdominal pain, or fever, call me sooner. Do you have any questions?	Srta. Ley, le vamos a hacer un examen serológico para confirmar el diagnóstico de embarazo. También le vamos a sacar sangre para ver cómo andan su hemoglobina y su hematocrito. Algunas veces los niveles pueden ser bajos si usted pierde mucha sangre durante la menstruación. También es importante analizar el nivel de glucosa o azúcar en la sangre. También tenemos que hacerle un examen de orina para asegurarnos de que no haya proteínas o azúcar en la orina. Le vamos a hacer un ultrasonido en cuatro semanas. Me gustaría verla de nuevo en un mes. Si tiene algún problema antes de volver, como sangrado o flujo vaginal, retortijones *(cólicos)* en el estómago o fiebre, llámeme de inmediato. ¿Tiene alguna pregunta?	Srta. Ley, le vamos a hacer un examen para confirmar el embarazo. También le vamos a sacar sangre para ver cómo andan la hemoglobina y el hematocrito. A veces los niveles pueden ser bajos si pierde mucha sangre durante la regla. También tenemos que ver cómo está el nivel de glucosa o azúcar en la sangre. Además, tenemos que hacerle un examen de orina para estar seguros de que no tiene proteínas o azúcar en la orina. Dentro de 4 semanas le vamos a hacer un ultrasonido. Me gustaría verla de nuevo en un mes. Si tiene algún problema antes, como sangrado por la vagina o desecho, retortijones en la panza o calentura, llámeme de inmediato. ¿Tiene alguna pregunta?

Of importance here is to confirm the diagnosis of pregnancy and assure oneself this is a normal, uterine pregnancy. Our patient has all the clinical signs of pregnancy: nausea, breast engorgement, etc. However, laboratory confirmation is necessary. Always ask about prior pregnancies because problems such as gestational diabetes and preeclampsia or so-called toxemia of pregnancy often will present with problems during the first pregnancy.

Preeclampsia is defined by hypertension and proteinuria. It is unusual to see this complication prior to 20 weeks gestation. If the disease progresses to seizures, then it is termed eclampsia. It is the second leading cause of maternal mortality and is responsible for significant fetal morbidity and mortality due to the high risk of premature birth. In mild cases, only hypertension and proteinuria are present; however, in severe cases cerebral edema, visual disturbances, liver dysfunction, and DIC may develop, creating a life-threatening situation. Risk factors include younger age and family history. Treatment initially is focused on control of the elevated blood pressure and anti-convulsive therapy. If severe symptoms develop, delivery of the fetus may be the only definitive option.

Gestational diabetes is a common complication that may occur during pregnancy. It is definitively diagnosed by a 3-hour oral glucose tolerance test, but may be suspected when glucose is present in the urine or fasting blood glucose is elevated. Major complications may result from gestational diabetes including preeclampsia hypertension and need for cesarean section to deliver the baby. The infant is also at risk for hypoglycemia, hypocalcemia, and macrosomia, birth trauma due to the large size of the infant. In addition, studies suggest an increased risk in the infants later on for childhood obesity. Treatment consists of nutritional counseling initially. Insulin therapy may be required to control the glucose level.

VOCABULARY

English	Español
Abortion	Aborto, aborto provocado, aborto quirúrgico
Abscess	Absceso
Adnexa	Anexos (trompas de Falopio, ovarios, ligamentos, etc.)
Birth control pills	Pastillas para evitar el embarazo, patillas anticonceptivas
Birth control, contraception	Métodos anticonceptivos, métodos para prevenir el embarazo
Bloated	Empanzado, con el estómago hinchado, lleno
Blood count	Conteo de células de la sangre, glóbulos rojos, hemograma
Breast	Seno, pecho, busto, mama, teta, chichi
Bruise	Magulladura, moretón, mancha
Cancer stage	Estadio del cáncer, etapa
Cervix	Cuello de la matriz, cérviz, cuello uterino
Clot	Coágulo, trombo
Colposcopy	Colposcopía
Condoms	Condones, profilácticos
Cul-de-sac	Fondo de saco
Cyst of ovary	Quiste de ovario
Chills	Escalofríos, calofríos
Dilation and curettage	Legrado, dilatación y curetaje, raspado de la matriz
Ectopic pregnancy	Embarazo ectópico
Fallopian tubes	Trompas de Falopio, tubos
Glove	Guante
Gynecologic diseases	Enfermedades ginecológicas, enfermedades del aparato reproductivo
Gynecologist	Ginecólogo, especialista de ginecología

English	Español
Having sex, sexual relations	Relaciones sexuales, tener relaciones, tener sexo
Heavy bleeding	Sangrado abundante, mucho sangrado
Hot flashes	Bochorno, calores
Hysterectomy	Operación para quitar la matriz o útero, histerectomía
Infertility	Esterilidad, cuando el hombre no puede fecundar ni la mujer puede concebir, infertilidad
Intrauterine device (IUD)	Dispositivo intrauterino (DIU)
Menopause	Menopausia, climaterio
Menstrual period	Regla, menstruación, período menstrual
Miscarriage	Pérdida, aborto espontáneo
Neonatology	Servicio de recién nacidos, neonatología
Obstetrician	Obstetra, especialista en obstetricia
Outpatient clinic	Consulta externa, clínica de consulta externa
PAP smear	Examen de Papanicolau
Pelvic exam	Examen pélvico, examen vaginal
Pelvic inflammatory disease (PID)	Enfermedad pélvica inflamatoria
Polyp	Pólipo
Pregnancy test	Prueba de embarazo
Sanitary pads	Toallas sanitarias, toallas femeninas
Sexual partner	Compañero sexual, pareja sexual, pareja
Sexually transmitted infection (STI)	Infección de transmisión sexual (ITS)
Speculum	Espéculo
Spotting	Manchado, manchas de sangre en la toalla sanitaria
Stillbirth	Bebé o feto que nace muerto, mortinato
Tampons	Tampones
Tubal ligation	Amarrar los tubos, ligar las trompas de Falopio, salpingectomía
Twisted ovary	Torsión de ovario
Unprotected sex	Relaciones sexuales sin protección, sexo sin protección, relaciones sin condón
Uterus	Útero, matriz
Vaginal discharge	Desecho, flujo o secreción por la vagina (vaginal)
Vaginal bleeding	Sangrado vaginal, sangrado por la vagina
Venereal disease	Enfermedad venérea, enfermedad de transmisión sexual
Yeast infection	Candidiasis vaginal

GRAMMATICAL TIPS

DIRECT OBJECT PRONOUNS

When listening, speaking, or practicing Spanish, you will notice that direct object pronouns and indirect object pronouns are used all over the place. In this chapter, you will be exposed to them and the following is an introduction to these pronouns.

The object that directly receives the action of the verb is called the direct object. It answers the question whom? *(¿A quién?)* or what? *(¿Qué?)* in relation to the sentence's subject and verb.

Direct object pronouns:

me (me)
te (you—familiar)
lo, la (him, her, it, you—formal)
nos (us)
los, las (them, you all—formal)

Always place it **before** the conjugated verb:

*Julio llama **a su madre.***	*Julio **la** llama.*
(¿A quién?)	
Julio calls his mother.	Julio calls her.

Commands (attach it at the end and add an accent for stress or emphasis):

*Manda **la carta**.* (= Send the letter.)
Mándala. (= Send it.)

Negative Sentences

In negative sentences, place *no* in front of the pronoun.
Examples:

No compro los libros. (= I don't buy the books.)
*No **los** compro.* (= I don't buy them.)

Direct object pronouns used with an infinitive or a present participle should be placed before the conjugated verb or attached to the infinitive or the present participle. (A written accent is needed to retain the stressed vowel of a present participle when a direct pronoun is attached to the end.)
Examples:

A. ***Lo*** *voy a comprar.*
B. *Voy a comprar**lo.***

A. ***Lo*** *estoy comprando.*
B. *Estoy comprándo**lo**.*

With reflexive verbs in the infinitive form, the direct object pronoun is placed after the reflexive verb at the end of the verb.
Examples:

Voy a probarme el suéter.
Voy a probármelo.

INDIRECT OBJECT PRONOUNS

The indirect object tells us where the direct object is going:

me = to/for me	*nos* = to/for us
te = to/for you (informal)	
le = to/for you (formal), him, her	*les* = to/for you (formal in Spain), them

Indirect objects (and their respective pronouns) refer to people already mentioned as indirect objects; that is, the pronoun tells to whom (*¿A quién?*) or for whom (*¿Para quién?*) the action of the verb is performed.

The indirect object pronouns are placed in the same position as direct object pronouns.

Direct and Indirect Object Pronouns Used Together

Sentences that have an indirect object usually also have a direct object. Remember, the indirect object pronoun tells us where the direct object pronoun is going. Notice how the sentences below just wouldn't work without a direct object.

Examples:

Él da a María el libro, la pluma (He gives María the book, the pen)
Él me compra flores, dulces, etc. (He buys me flowers, candy, etc.)

When you have both a *direct object pronoun* and an *indirect object pronoun* in the same sentence, the *indirect object* pronoun comes first.

Indirect Object

Le and *les* always change to *se* when they are used together with the direct object pronouns: *lo, la, los, las.*

The reason for such changes is because *le lo* sounds like a tongue-twister and it is easier to pronounce *se lo.*

le lo = *se lo*
le la = *se la*
le los = *se los*
le las = *se las*
les lo = *se lo*
les la = *se la*
les los = *se los*
les las = *se las*

Double Object Pronouns

*El doctor quita **la calentura al paciente.***

Direct Object Pronoun (*la,*) Indirect Object Pronoun (*le*)

*El doctor **se la** quita.* (change *le* to *se*) (= The doctor takes it from him.)
What? From whom? He takes the fever away from the patient.

La enfermera me da la pastilla a mí. (= The nurse gives the pill to me.)
*La enfermera **me la** da.*

Negative Sentences

In negative sentences, the negative word comes directly before the first pronoun.

No se la quito. (I don't take it away from him.)
No me la quites. (Don't take it away from me.)

In sentences with a verb followed by an infinitive, there are two options regarding the placement of the pronouns. Place them immediately before the conjugated verb or attach them directly to the verb in the infinitive.

El enfermero quiere hacer el ultrasonido a Jorge.
A. *El enfermero **se lo** quiere hacer.*
B. *El enfermero quiere hacér**selo**.*

Double Object Pronouns with Commands

Attach them to the end of the command and write an accent mark (specify where you place the accent mark).

*¡Toma **la presión a Pedro!***

Indirect Object Pronoun, *la*; Indirect Object Pronoun, *le*

*¡Tóma**sela**!* (Take it!)

*Da me **la píldora a mí.***(Give the pill to me.)

*¡Dá**mela**!* (Give it to me!)

Negative Commands

Place them before the command and after *no*:

No **me la** tomes.
No **me la** des.

EJERCICIO:

Ahora vamos a practicar.

1. La madre le lee **el libro al niño**. Ella _____ lee.

2. Marta **te** enseña **las fotos**. Marta_____ enseña.

3. Sara les vende **la moto a sus amigos**. Sara_____ vende.

4. Ella **nos** sirve **unos tequilas**. Ella_____ sirve.

5. Sofía **me** compra **unos sellos**. Sofía _____ compra.

6. Lola les pide **a Uds. un favor grande**. Lola_____ pide.

7. Tú y yo le damos **cien dólares a Luis**. Tú y yo_____ damos.

8. Tu padre **te** paga **las cuentas**. Tu padre_____ paga.

9. Ellos **nos** dicen **un chiste bueno**. Ellos_____ dicen.

10. Mis tíos **me muestran una foto**. Mis tíos_____ muestran.

CULTURAL TIPS: LA *MOLLERA CAÍDA*

La *mollera caída* is another illness that is supposed to have an effect on children. It is related to the soft spot on the head of a newborn child. When a baby becomes dehydrated, the soft spot is felt as deep. The baby will show symptoms of dehydration. However, in some instances families will try home remedies and take the baby to a *curandero(a)* or an elder and they will try to lift the fallen soft spot. They will introduce the middle or index finger in the baby's mouth and try to lift the soft spot from the pallet. It is believed that the soft spot falls because of mishandling the baby or evil eye. Evil eye happens when someone feels like touching a baby and they do not dare to. Energy, negative because of the desire to caress the baby is not satisfied, is transmitted. When a pregnant woman does not let people touch her stomach, evil eye is produced as well. To prevent evil eye, some people will safety pin a seed called deer eye to the baby's clothes or to themselves if they are pregnant. This seed is believed to have the power to reflect evil eye and therefore it protects the person.

5 Urologic Diseases

INTRODUCTION

ANATOMY

Figure 5-1 illustrates the anatomy of the urologic system.

KIDNEY STONES

Pain is the most common symptom in patients presenting with renal stones. It can be quite variable in severity and location depending upon the location of the stone in the renal collecting system and the size of the stone. Stones located in the upper ureter and renal pelvis may present with abdominal and flank pain, often radiating into the groin. As the stone passes to a lower location, it is typically a lower abdominal, groin, and testicular pain that is experienced. Remember this is a visceral pain with irritation and obstruction of the ureter, thus the pain is often poorly localized. In most patients it is severe; however, it may be quite mild depending on the degree of spasm of the ureter and the degree of obstruction. Patients may also have asymptomatic stones discovered when radiographs are performed for other reasons. Most asymptomatic stones are located in the renal pelvis, whereas symptoms usually become present as the stone moves into the ureter. Gross hematuria may be noted by the patient, but more often it is microscopic and diagnosed by urine analysis, the exam performed when a stone is suspected.

There are many risk factors for kidney stones. Most stones in the United States are calcium stones. Thus, any factor that increases calcium in the urine will predispose to stone formation. Uric acid stones account for about 10% of stones and usually occur in patients without underlying disease. They are obviously more common in patients with increased urine uric acid, as occurs in gout.

Diagnosis of renal stones is made by a good clinical history followed by physical exam. With confirmatory tests, the diagnosis is made with certainty and treated. The following is a typical case presentation of a patient with a kidney stone.

Figure 5-1. Anatomy of the urologic system in English and Spanish.

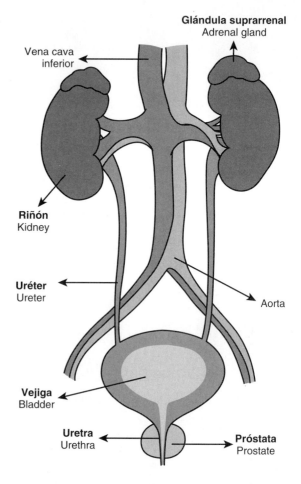

Glándula suprarrenal
Adrenal gland

Vena cava
inferior

Riñón
Kidney

Uréter
Ureter

Aorta

Vejiga
Bladder

Uretra
Urethra

Próstata
Prostate

CASE 1: KIDNEY STONE

CHIEF COMPLAINT

Mr. Adams is a 23-year-old construction worker in Arizona who presents to your clinic with excruciating right lower quadrant abdominal and right flank pain.

HISTORY

	English	Spanish Formal	Spanish Informal
Q.	Hello, Mr. Adams. My name is Dr. Sullivan. What brings you to see us today?	Hola, Sr. Adams. Mi nombre es Dra. Sullivan. ¿Por qué viene a vernos el día de hoy?	Hola, Sr. Adams, soy la Dra. Sullivan. ¿Por qué viene a visitarnos hoy?
A.	Hi, Doctor. I have a pain that is killing me in my stomach.	Hola, doctora. Tengo un dolor de estómago que me está matando.	Tengo mucho dolor de estómago.
Q.	Where is it located?	¿Dónde es el dolor?	¿Dónde le duele?
A.	Lower down on the right side of my stomach and my back.	En la parte de abajo, en el lado derecho del estómago y la espalda.	Abajo, en el lado derecho del estómago y la espalda.

	English	Spanish Formal	Spanish Informal
Q.	Can you point to the areas where it hurts?	¿Me puede enseñar el área donde le duele?	Enséñeme donde le duele.
A.	(Patient points to the right lower abdomen and groin and right flank.)	(Paciente señala el abdomen inferior derecho, la ingle y el flanco derecho.)	Aquí. (El paciente señala el abdomen inferior derecho, la ingle y el flanco derecho.)
Q.	On a scale of 1 to 10, how would you rate the pain, 10 being the worst pain you have ever had?	En una escala de uno a diez, donde diez es el peor dolor que usted ha tenido en su vida, ¿cómo clasificaría (catalogaría) este dolor?	De uno a diez, en donde diez es el peor dolor que ha tenido, ¿cómo diría usted que es este dolor?
A.	It is about an eight or nine.	Es como un ocho o un nueve.	Como ocho o nueve.
Q.	When did it start?	¿Cuándo le comenzó?	¿Cuándo empezó?
A.	It began this morning about 9 or 10 o'clock.	Me comenzó esta mañana, como a las nueve o diez.	En la mañana, como a las nueve o diez.
Q.	Is it getting worse?	¿Está empeorando?	¿Es peor ahora que antes?
A.	Yes, this morning it was an ache, but now it hurts really badly.	Sí, esta mañana era sólo un poco (leve), pero ahora me duele mucho (muy intenso).	Sí, en la mañana era un poco, pero ahora duele mucho.
Q.	How would you describe the pain? In other words, is it sharp or dull?	¿Cómo describiría el dolor? O en otras palabras, ¿es agudo (punzante) o sordo?	¿Cómo es el dolor? ¿Agudo o sordo?
A.	It is dull and achy.	Es sordo y doloroso.	Es un dolor sordo.
Q.	Does it move anywhere?	¿Se mueve para alguna otra parte del cuerpo?	¿Se mueve para algún lugar?
A.	Yes. It moves to my groin and a testicle.	Sí, se mueve para la ingle y el testículo.	Sí, para la ingle y el testículo.
Q.	Does it come and go or is it constant?	¿Es constante o viene y se va?	¿Lo tiene todo el tiempo o le pega y se le quita?
A.	At first, it would come and go, but for the past hour or so it is constant.	Al principio, venía y se iba pero en la última hora ha sido constante.	Antes me pegaba y se me quitaba, pero ahora es todo el tiempo.
Q.	What makes it better or worse?	¿Qué lo hace mejor o peor?	¿Qué mejora o empeora el dolor?
A.	Nothing really helps. I cannot get comfortable.	Realmente, nada me ayuda. No me puedo sentir cómodo.	Nada me lo quita. Nada me hace sentir bien.
Q.	Does it hurt more if you move than if you stay still?	¿Duele más cuando se mueve que cuando se queda quieto?	¿Le duele más si se mueve?
A.	No, in fact I can't sit still because of the pain.	No, de hecho no me puedo sentar quieto por el dolor.	No. No me puedo sentar sin moverme por el dolor.
Q.	Have you had any problems urinating, such as burning or the feeling of urgency to urinate?	¿Ha tenido algún problema para orinar, como ardor o sensación de urgencia?	¿Ha tenido algún problema para orinar, como quemazón o como sentir que si no va inmediatamente se va a orinar?
A.	Yes. I feel the need to urinate but nothing comes out except a few drops of urine. I have not had any burning.	Sí, siento la necesidad de orinar, pero nada me sale, sólo unas gotas. No he sentido ardor al orinar.	Sí, siento la necesidad de orinar, pero nada me sale, sólo unas gotitas. No he sentido quemazón.
Q.	Have you ever passed a kidney stone before?	¿Alguna vez ha orinado un cálculo o piedra del riñón?	¿Alguna vez le ha salido una piedra del riñón por la orina?
A.	No. Not that I know of.	No. No que yo sepa.	No.
Q.	Have you had any nausea or vomiting?	¿Ha tenido náusea o vómito?	¿Ha tenido ganas de vomitar o vomitó?
A.	Yes. I felt nauseated since this morning and vomited twice before arriving at the hospital.	Sí. He sentido náuseas desde la mañana y vomité dos veces antes de llegar al hospital.	Sí. He tenido ganas de vomitar desde la mañana y vomité dos veces.

	English	Spanish Formal	Spanish Informal Continued
Q.	Do you suffer from any medical illnesses such as heart or lung disease?	¿Padece de alguna enfermedad, como del corazón o los pulmones?	¿Padece del corazón o de los pulmones?
A.	No.	No.	No.
Q.	Is there any history of abdominal problems?	¿Alguna vez ha tenido problemas del estómago?	¿Ha padecido de problemas de la panza alguna vez?
A.	My doctor once told me I had acid reflux and gave me medication to reduce the acid.	Mi doctor me dijo una vez que tenía reflujo y me dio un medicamento para disminuir el ácido.	Una vez el doctor me dijo que tenía reflujo y me dio unas medicinas para bajar el ácido.
Q.	Have you ever had surgery?	¿Le han hecho cirugía alguna vez?	¿Alguna vez lo han operado?
A.	Yes. I had my appendix out at six years of age.	Sí. Me quitaron el apéndice cuando tenía seis años.	Sí, me sacaron el apéndice cuando tenía seis años.
Q.	Are you taking any medications?	¿Está tomando alguna medicina?	¿Y toma alguna medicina?
A.	I have been taking ibuprofen for a strained knee.	He estado tomando ibuprofen para una rodilla que se me torció (dislocó).	Estoy tomando ibuprofen para la torcedura de la rodilla.
Q.	Do you have any allergies to medications?	¿Padece de alergias a alguna medicina?	¿Es alérgico a alguna medicina?
A.	No.	No.	No.
Q.	Do you smoke cigarettes, drink alcohol, or use drugs?	¿Fuma cigarrillos, toma licor o usa drogas?	¿Toma licor, fuma cigarrillos o usa drogas?
A.	I used to smoke cigarettes but gave them up two years ago. I drink once in a while at parties, but only a beer or two.	Fumaba cigarrillos, pero los dejé hace dos años. Tomo de vez en cuando en las fiestas pero sólo una o dos cervezas.	Fumaba, pero lo dejé hace dos años. Tomo de vez en cuando, pero sólo una o dos cervezas.
Q.	Mr. Adams, can you please change into a gown? I will return. Please remove your underwear too. First I am going to listen to your heart and lungs. I am also going to examine your stomach and back. Mr. Adams, I need to do an exam of your groin and testicles to see if there is a hernia or a problem in the testicle that is giving you pain. Finally, I need to do a rectal exam to check your prostate because sometimes infection in the prostate can give some of the symptoms you have.	Sr. Adams, ¿se puede poner una bata, por favor? Yo regresaré pronto. Por favor, quítese la ropa interior también. Primero le voy a escuchar el corazón y los pulmones. También le voy a examinar el estómago y la espalda. Sr. Adams, necesito examinarle la ingle y los testículos para ver si hay una hernia o un problema en los testículos que está causando el dolor. Finalmente, necesito hacerle un tacto rectal para examinar la próstata porque a veces las infecciones de la próstata pueden causar algunos de los síntomas que tiene.	Sr. Adams, ¿se puede poner una bata, por favor? Quítese la ropa interior, yo regresaré pronto. Le voy a oír el corazón y los pulmones. Después le voy a examinar el estómago y la espalda. Sr. Adams, tengo que examinarle la ingle y los testículos para ver si tiene una hernia o algún problema de los testículos que está causando el dolor. Finalmente, necesito hacerle un tacto rectal para revisar la próstata porque a veces las infecciones de la próstata pueden causar los síntomas que tiene usted.

PHYSICAL EXAM

Vital signs: BP 130/90, P 110, Temp. 37.4°C, RR 16
    Pertinent findings:

- **Chest**: Clear to auscultation.
- **Heart**: Tachycardia, normal rhythm, no murmurs, no S3 or S4.

- **Abdominal exam**: Diffuse tenderness in the right lower abdomen. There is no involuntary guarding present. Mild voluntary guarding is present in the right lower quadrant.
- **Back**: There is significant right flank tenderness present.
- **Genito-urinary**: There are no hernias, testicles are normal size, non-tender, without masses.
- **Rectal**: Prostate is normal size, uniform without masses, and non-tender, no masses are palpated in the rectum and the stool is guiac negative.

This is a fairly classic presentation for a kidney stone. Despite this, we still need to form a differential diagnosis. The intensity of the pain, the location, and quality are very classic for a renal stone. The pain tends to be dull and poorly localized due to the visceral nerve path of the pain; thus there is no involuntary guarding like we would see in the acute peritoneal inflammation of advanced appendicitis. The flank tenderness that is elicited by gently hitting the flank region with the closed hand or heel of the palm is consistent with a urologic problem. Remember, the urologic system is retroperitoneal; thus urinary problems such as stones and infection often present with back pain. In the differential diagnosis, appendicitis has to be listed. The presentation is highly unusual. The fact that our patient states he had his appendix removed as a child makes this diagnosis very unlikely (the patient may think that he had an appendectomy as a child, but in reality the surgeon found other pathology and did not remove the appendix; or, as rarely occurs, the appendix may have been removed but the base of the appendix was left, making it possible for the patient to develop appendicitis again). In a female, one would want to rule out ectopic pregnancy and tubo-ovarian pathology such as torsion of the ovary, which is sudden and may present with severe pain. Inguinal hernia with incarceration (entrapment of intra-abdominal contents in the hernia sac) may present with the above symptoms, making it imperative to do a careful hernia exam. Finally, testicular disease such as epididymitis, an inflammation of the testicular epididymis, may present with similar pain, but the greatest pain to palpation would be on the posterior part of the testicle. Prostatitis, an infection of the prostate, likewise may present with mainly urinary symptoms such as urgency and frequency of urination and severe tenderness on rectal exam. Often fever is present.

To confirm the diagnosis of a kidney stone, an initial urine analysis is very helpful. Over 90% of patients with kidney stones will have hematuria on microscopic examination of urine sample. However, the absence of hematuria doesn't rule out a stone but would make the diagnosis less likely. A non-contrast, helical CT scan is the procedure of choice for confirming the diagnosis of a stone. It is also predictive for the spontaneous passage of stones, which depends on the size of the stone. Those less than 4 mm have a very high rate of passage, while this decreases with increasing diameter of the stone. If a stone fails to pass, endoscopic intervention is often required.

FOLLOW-UP

	English	Spanish Formal	Spanish Informal
Q.	Mr. Adams, I believe you have a kidney stone. The first priority is to get your pain under control. The nurse will be in to start	Sr. Adams, yo creo que usted tiene un cálculo en el riñón. La prioridad es controlar el dolor. La enfermera le va a poner un suero	Sr. Adams, creo que tiene una piedra en el riñón. La prioridad es quitarle el dolor. La enfermera le va a poner un

	English	Spanish Formal	Spanish Informal Continued
	an intravenous and give you fluid and pain medicine through your vein. The next step is to get a sample of urine from you to check for blood. A CT scan will confirm the diagnosis of a stone and will rule out other possibilities for the pain you have. Most people pass the stone and go home. Occasionally, if the stone is large, we may have to admit you to the hospital and the urologists may have to remove it. By giving you a large amount of fluid through the vein, more urine will be produced, helping to wash away the kidney stone. The fact that you have vomited may result in dehydration and lowered urinary output. Do you have any questions?	intravenoso para darle líquido y medicina para el dolor por la vena. El próximo paso es tomar una muestra de orina para ver si tiene sangre. Una tomografía nos ayudará a confirmar el diagnóstico de un cálculo y a descartar otras causas de dolor. La mayoría de las personas expulsan la piedra y se van para la casa. De vez en cuando, si la piedra es grande, es posible que haya que internar a la persona en el hospital para que un urólogo se la saque. Le vamos a dar una gran cantidad de líquido por la vena para que orine más y expulse la piedra con la orina. Como ha vomitado, existe la posibilidad de que se deshidrate y orine menor cantidad. ¿Tiene alguna pregunta?	suero por la vena para darle líquidos y un analgésico para el dolor. Lo que sigue es tomar una muestra de orina para ver si hay sangre. Una tomografía nos ayudará a confirmar que existe una piedra y descartar otras causas de dolor. Generalmente, las personas botan la piedra y se van para la casa. De vez en cuando, si la piedra es grande, hay que internarlas en el hospital para que el urólogo se la saque. Le vamos a dar muchos líquidos por la vena para que orine más y bote la piedra. Como ha vomitado, se puede deshidratar y orinar menos. ¿Tiene preguntas?
A.	Yes. How did I get the stone, and will it happen again?	Sí. ¿Cómo se formó el cálculo? Y ¿es posible que se vuelva a formar?	Sí. ¿Cómo se forman las piedras? Y ¿es posible que se vuelvan a formar?
Q.	In most people no cause is found. In your case, being a construction worker, you are out in the sun and here in Arizona it is hot. Dehydration is a very common predisposing factor in healthy people to form stones. If this is the case you will need to drink plenty of fluid while working. When you go home you will be given a strainer to strain your urine for stones. You should save the stone so that your doctor can do an analysis on it to see what it is made up of. In this way they can determine if any other tests should be done. Do you have any other questions?	En la mayoría de los casos no sabemos cómo se forman. En su caso, como trabaja en construcción y pasa una gran parte del tiempo expuesto al sol, y aquí en Arizona es caliente, la deshidratación es un factor muy común que predispone a las personas para que formen piedras en los riñones. Si éste es el caso, usted va a tener que tomar muchos líquidos cuando está trabajando. Le vamos a dar un colador para que se lo lleve a su casa y cuele la orina para ver si expulsa la piedra. Si la piedra sale, tiene que guardarla para que la analice el doctor y vea de qué está compuesta. De esta manera, ellos pueden determinar si hay que hacer algún otro examen. ¿Tiene alguna pregunta?	Generalmente, no sabemos cómo se forman. En su caso, como trabaja en construcción y pasa mucho tiempo al sol, y aquí es muy caliente, es posible que la deshidratación sea un factor que predispone a que se formen piedras en los riñones. Si es así, debería tomar mucha agua y refrescos cuando esté trabajando. Le vamos a dar un colador para que cuele la orina en su casa y se dé cuenta cuando bote la piedra. Si la piedra sale, tiene que guardarla para que la vea el doctor. De esta manera, ellos pueden saber si hay que hacer algún otro examen. ¿Tiene alguna otra pregunta?
A.	No. I understand things very well.	No. Entiendo muy bien lo que me dijo.	No.

TEST RESULTS

The following is the result of our tests.

- Urine analysis 4+ blood
- 20 to 30 red blood cells (RBC)/HPF
- CT scan (Fig. 5-2) reveals a 4-mm stone in the left ureter with proximal ureteral dilation.

Both confirm the diagnosis of a renal stone. The fact that it is less than 5 mm in diameter makes spontaneous passage very likely.

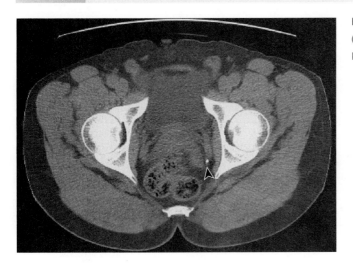

Figure 5-2. CT scan demonstrating a kidney stone in the ureter. (From Townsend C: *Sabiston Textbook of Surgery*, ed 17. Philadelphia, WB Saunders, 2004.)

CASE 2: URINARY TRACT INFECTION

An extremely common problem seen in clinical practice is urinary tract infection. In both the adult population and the pediatric age group, this is a commonly seen problem. The clinical presentation ranges from minimal symptomatology to full-blown septic shock. Most urinary tract infections result from bacteria that enter through the urethra and ascend to the bladder. Thus, urinary tract infection is much more common in the female patient than the male, due to the short urethra in the former. In fact, in the pediatric patient a urinary tract infection that occurs in the male is often the result of a congenital anatomic defect such as incompetent valves at the uretero-vesical junction, allowing reflux of urine. In the female child, however, urinary tract infection is fairly common due to the proximity of the urethra and rectum and the short distance from the urethra to the bladder. In fact, in the male patient, a single-time urinary tract infection warrants a workup to evaluate the urologic system. In the female patient, a workup is only done after repeated infections.

The clinical presentation of a urinary tract infection is variable, but most patients have pain and burning on urination, termed dysuria. In addition, due to the irritation of the urethra, urgency—the sensation that one has to urinate—is often present although little urine may be present in the urinary bladder. Frequency of urination is present as well. Fever may or may not be present depending on the location of the infection. If the infection is confined to the urinary bladder (cystitis), then fever may be low grade or absent. If, however, the infection ascends to the kidney (pyelonephritis), then high fever and shaking chills may be present as well as nausea and vomiting. The latter may be life-threatening if not treated urgently. With urinary tract infection, pain is often present but is much milder than that seen with kidney stones. With bladder infections, the most common site of urinary tract infection, often there is mild pain in the suprapubic region but pain may be absent. When infection ascends to involve the kidney, the pain becomes much more intense due to inflammation and stretching of the renal capsule, which is richly innervated. In this case, patients complain of moderate to severe upper abdominal and flank pain.

The following is a common presentation of the above clinical problem.

CHIEF COMPLAINT

Miss Soto is a 21-year-old female who presents with burning on urination and mild lower abdominal pain.

HISTORY

	English	Spanish Formal	Spanish Informal
Q.	Hello, Ms. Soto, my name is Bob Belsher. I am a fourth-year medical student working with Dr. James. I am going to ask you some questions and then Dr. James will be in.	Hola, Srta. Soto, mi nombre es Bob Belsher. Soy estudiante de medicina de cuarto año. Trabajo con el Dr. James. Le voy a hacer unas preguntas y después vendrá el Dr. James.	Hola, Srta. Soto, me llamo Bob Belsher. Soy estudiante de medicina de cuarto año. Trabajo con el Dr. James. Le voy a hacer unas preguntas antes de que venga el Dr. James.
A.	That's fine, please call me Christina.	Está bien, por favor llámeme Christina.	Bien, me puede llamar Christina.
Q.	Okay. Christina, what brings you in today to see us?	Está bien. Christina, ¿por qué viene a vernos hoy?	Está bien. ¿Por qué viene hoy?
A.	For the past five or six days I have had burning when I urinate.	Los últimos cinco o seis días he tenido ardor al orinar.	He tenido quemazón al orinar los últimos cinco o seis días.
Q.	Is it getting better or worse?	¿Está mejor o peor que cuando comenzó?	¿Está empeorando o mejorando?
A.	It is getting worse, especially over the past two days.	Está peor, especialmente en los últimos dos días.	Está empeorado, especialmente los últimos dos días.
Q.	Do you have pain on urination?	¿Tiene dolor al orinar?	¿Le duele cuando orina?
A.	Yes. For the last day it hurts when I urinate.	Sí. He tenido dolor al orinar desde ayer.	Sí. Me ha dolido al orinar desde ayer.
Q.	Do you have to urinate more often?	¿Tiene que orinar con más frecuencia?	¿Está orinando con más frecuencia?
A.	Yes. I feel like I have to go to the bathroom all the time.	Sí. Siento ganas de ir al baño todo el tiempo.	Sí. Me dan ganas de orinar a toda hora.
Q.	Does the usual amount of urine come out when you go to the bathroom?	Cuando va al baño, ¿orina la misma cantidad de orina que siempre?	Cuando orina, ¿le sale la misma cantidad de orina que lo normal?
A.	No, very little comes out.	No, orino muy poco.	No, sale muy poco, sólo unas gotas.
Q.	Have you had any stomach pain?	¿Ha tenido dolor de estómago?	¿Le ha dolido el estómago?
A.	Yes, for the past day I have had pain in the lower part of my stomach.	Sí, he tenido dolor en la parte de abajo del estómago desde ayer.	Sí, desde ayer me ha dolido la parte de abajo del estómago.
Q.	Is there any chance you might be pregnant?	¿Es posible que usted este embarazada?	¿Podría estar embarazada?
A.	No, I had my last period three days ago.	No, tuve mi última regla hace tres días.	No, tuve la regla hace tres días.
Q.	Have you had any back pain?	¿Ha tenido dolor de espalda?	¿Le ha dolido la espalda?
A.	No, I have had no back pain.	No, no he tenido dolor de espalda.	No.

	English	Spanish Formal	Spanish Informal
Q.	Have you had any fever or chills?	¿Ha tenido fiebre o escalofríos?	¿Le ha dado calentura o escalofríos?
A.	No. I haven't taken my temperature but I haven't felt warm.	No. No me he tomado la temperatura pero no me he sentido afiebrada.	No.
Q.	Have you had any nausea or vomiting?	¿Ha tenido náusea o vómito?	¿Ha tenido ganas de vomitar o ha vomitado?
A.	No, I have had a good appetite.	No, he tenido buen apetito.	No, tengo buen apetito.
Q.	Have you ever had a urinary tract infection before?	¿Alguna vez ha tenido una infección de las vías urinarias?	¿Alguna vez ha tenido infección de orina?
A.	I think when I was a child I did.	Creo que tuve una infección cuando era niña.	Creo que sí, cuando era pequeña.
Q.	Christina, I need to ask some personal questions that are related to the symptoms you have.	Christina, necesito hacerle unas preguntas personales que están relacionadas con sus síntomas.	Christina, tengo que hacerle unas preguntas personales que tienen que ver con los síntomas que tiene.
A.	Fine.	Bien.	Está bien.
Q.	Have you had any vaginal discharge other than your recent period?	¿Ha tenido algún flujo o secreción vaginal además de la regla?	Aparte de la regla, ¿ha tenido algún desecho por la vagina?
A.	No, I have had no vaginal discharge.	No, no he tenido flujo por la vagina.	No.
Q.	Are you active sexually?	¿Está activa sexualmente?	¿Está teniendo relaciones sexuales regularmente?
A.	Yes, I have a boyfriend.	Sí, tengo un novio.	Sí, tengo novio.
Q.	Do you use any form of birth control?	¿Usa algún método anticonceptivo?	¿Usa algún método para evitar el embarazo?
A.	Yes, my boyfriend uses a condom.	Sí, mi novio usa un condón.	Sí, mi novio usa un condón.
Q.	Do you have more than one partner?	¿Tiene más de una pareja?	¿Tiene más de un compañero sexual?
A.	No. My boyfriend and I have been together for the past three years.	No, mi novio y yo hemos estado juntos los últimos tres años.	No, he estado con mi novio por tres años.
Q.	Do you have any medical illnesses such as heart or lung disease?	¿Tiene alguna enfermedad, como del corazón o los pulmones?	¿Padece de alguna enfermedad, como del corazón o los pulmones?
A.	No. I am in good health.	No, tengo buena salud.	No, estoy bien.
Q.	Are you taking any medications?	¿Tomo algún medicamento?	¿Esta tomando alguna medicine?
A.	I take ibuprofen for menstrual cramping during my period.	Tomo ibuprofen para los calambres menstruales durante el período.	Tomo ibuprofen para los cólicos cuando tengo la regla.
Q.	Do you have any allergies to medications?	¿Tiene alguna alergia a los medicamentos?	¿Padece de alguna alergia a las medicinas?
A.	I broke out in a rash once when they gave me ampicillin.	Me broté con sarpullido una vez cuando me dieron ampicilina.	Me broté con ronchas una vez cuando me dieron ampicilina.
Q.	Christina, I am going to give you a gown to change into and I will be back with Dr. James. Do you have any questions so far?	Christina, le voy a dar una bata para que se cambie, y volveré con el Dr. James. ¿Tiene alguna pregunta hasta ahora?	Christina, le voy a dar una bata para que se cambie, y volveré con el Dr. James. ¿Tiene alguna pregunta?
A.	What do you think I have?	¿Qué cree usted que tengo?	¿Qué piensas que tengo?

	English	Spanish Formal	Spanish Informal Continued
Q.	I think you have a urinary tract infection, which is common at your age; however, the physical exam and certain simple tests such as a urine analysis and culture will confirm this. Dr. James will want to ask you some questions also and he might have a different opinion. I will be right back.	Yo creo que tiene una infección de las vías urinarias, lo que es común a su edad; sin embargo, el examen físico y ciertos exámenes sencillos, como un análisis de orina y un cultivo, lo van a confirmar. El Dr. James va a querer hacerle algunas preguntas también, y puede tener una opinión diferente. Volveré en un momento.	Yo creo que tiene una infección de orina, lo que es común a esta edad; sin embargo, el examen físico y otros exámenes sencillos, como un análisis de orina y un cultivo, lo van a confirmar. El Dr. James va a querer hacerle otras preguntas también, y puede tener otra opinión. Volveré en un momento.
A.	Thank you, Bob.	Gracias, Bob.	Gracias.

PHYSICAL EXAM

Vital signs: BP 110/70, P 64, RR 12, Temp. 37.2°C
  Pertinent physical findings:

- Abdominal exam: mild tenderness in the lower, central part of the abdomen. No voluntary or involuntary guarding. No flank tenderness.
- Pelvic exam not done.

DIFFERENTIAL DIAGNOSIS

The differential diagnosis is limited based on the age of the patient, the history, and the physical exam.

- Urinary tract infection (UTI) cystitis versus pylonephritis
- Ectopic pregnancy
- Acute salpingitis or pelvic inflammatory disease (PID)
- Appendicitis

Whether or not to do a pelvic exam is a clinical decision. If one is reasonably sure of the diagnosis of urinary tract infection, as in this case, the pelvic exam may be omitted. If one is considering a gynecologic problem, then a pelvic exam is crucial.

This is a classic presentation of a patient with a UTI. The initial complaint of dysuria keys you into that diagnosis, especially in a young female patient. As with any woman of childbearing age who presents with abdominal pain, one has to rule out ectopic pregnancy, a life-threatening event. The fact that her boyfriend uses a condom and her period was three days prior speaks against this; however, one still has to order a serum β-HCG to rule out pregnancy. Also much less likely is appendicitis, due to the location of the pain and the fact that she has a good appetite. One of the most consistent findings in appendicitis is anorexia. In fact, when a patient tells us he or she is hungry, appendicitis becomes much less likely, but one must still keep this diagnosis in mind. As one goes through medicine, there is a realization that it is rare for a patient to follow the "textbook" or classic presentation for appendicitis; thus, one must always consider diagnosis in the presence of lower abdominal pain. Salpingitis is also unlikely due to the fact that our patient has no vaginal discharge and the pain is mild. The pain of acute salpingitis or PID is usually severe. The fact that she has no back or flank pain is consistent with an infection confined to the bladder (cystitis) and not the kidney (pyelonephritis). Still, a careful physical exam is required to rule out all of the above diseases.

Labs: The key to the diagnosis of a UTI is the history and physical exam and a urine analysis and gram stain and culture. The analysis will confirm the diagnosis of UTI if over five white blood cells per high power field (HPF) and bacteria are present. The culture will take 24 to 48 hours for the bacteria to grow, so the initial diagnosis is confirmed by the analysis. It is also imperative to obtain a β-HCG for the reasons cited above.

CASE 3: BENIGN PROSTATIC HYPERTROPHY

Prostatic disease is a common cause of urinary problems in the older male patient. Typically, in the fifth decade of life the prostate begins to hypertrophy. Occasionally, the process starts earlier in the fourth decade and progresses. Since the prostate surrounds the urethra, urinary obstruction may occur with hypertrophy of the prostate, termed benign prostatic hypertrophy (BPH). This is a benign condition that may initially produce mild symptoms of urinary obstruction and progress slowly, sometimes over years. The following is an illustrative case.

CHIEF COMPLAINT

Mr. Ortiz, a 68-year-old male, presents to the emergency room with inability to urinate, fever, and severe lower abdominal pain.

HISTORY

	English	Spanish Formal	Spanish Informal
Q.	Hello, Mr. Ortiz, I am Anna Mann, a third year medical student working with Dr. Warneke. I am going to ask you some questions about your present illness and then Dr. Warneke will come in.	Hola, Sr. Ortiz, soy Anna Mann, estudiante de medicina de tercer año. Trabajo con el Dr. Warneke. Le voy a hacer algunas preguntas sobre su problema de salud y después el Dr. Warneke vendrá a verlo.	Hola, Sr. Ortiz, soy Anna Mann, estudiante de medicina de tercer año. Trabajo con el Dr. Warneke. Le voy a hacer unas preguntas y después vendrá a verlo el Dr. Warneke.
A.	That is fine, Anna.	Esta bien, Anna.	Está bien.
Q.	Why are you here today?	¿Por qué vino hoy?	¿Por qué vino a vernos?
A.	I can't urinate and my stomach is killing me.	No puedo orinar y el dolor de estómago me está matando.	No me sale la orina y tengo mucho dolor de estómago.
Q.	How old are you?	¿Qué edad tiene?	¿Cuántos años tiene?
A.	I am 68 years old.	Tengo sesenta y ocho años.	Sesenta y ocho años.
Q.	How long has it been since you urinated?	¿Cuándo fue la última vez que orinó?	¿Desde hace cuándo no orina?
A.	The last time I went to the bathroom was yesterday. It has been more than 12 hours.	Ayer fue la última vez que fui al baño. Hace más de doce horas.	La última vez fue ayer. Hace más de doce horas.

English	Spanish Formal	Spanish Informal	Continued
Q. Do you feel like you have to urinate?	¿Siente ganas de orinar?	¿Tiene ganas de orinar?	
A. Yes. I tried, but just a few drops of urine come out.	Sí. Traté de orinar, pero sólo me salieron unas gotas de orina.	Sí. Traté, pero sólo salieron unas gotas.	
Q. Have you had problems urinating before?	¿Ha tenido problemas para orinar antes?	¿Ha tenido problemas para orinar antes?	
A. Not this bad. Over the past year I have had problems urinating.	No tan mal. He tenido problemas para orinar el último año.	No tan mal. He tenido problemas para orinar todo el año.	
Q. Has the problem gotten worse?	¿Ha empeorado el problema?	¿Es peor ahora que al principio?	
A. Yes. It has gotten really bad over the past months.	Sí, ha empeorado los últimos meses.	Sí, se ha puesto peor en los últimos meses.	
Q. Do you have to strain to urinate?	¿Tiene que hacer fuerza para orinar?	¿Tiene que hacer fuerza para que le salga la orina?	
A. Yes. I have to push hard but not a lot comes out.	Sí. Tengo que empujar con fuerza pero casi no sale nada.	Sí, tengo que pujar recio pero casi nada sale.	
Q. Is the stream of urine weaker now than before?	¿Es el chorro de orina más débil que antes?	¿Es el chorro más débil que antes?	
A. Very much so.	Bastante.	Mucho más débil.	
Q. Is there a delay in starting the urinary stream?	¿Hay un atraso para que comience a salir el chorro?	¿Hay un atraso para comenzar a orinar?	
A. Yes. It sometimes takes a long time for the urine to come out. If I hold the urine in for a long time it makes it even worse.	Sí, a veces toma bastante tiempo para que salga la orina. Si sostengo la orina adentro por mucho tiempo, es aún peor.	Sí, a veces tarda mucho tiempo para que salga. Si la sostengo adentro por un rato, es peor.	
Q. Have you ever had to go to the hospital for that?	¿Alguna vez ha tenido que ir al hospital por este problema?	¿Alguna vez ha tenido que ir al hospital por esto?	
A. No. But there were times I thought I would have to go.	No. Pero a veces he pensado que debería de ir.	No. Pero a veces he creído que debería ir.	
Q. Have you had any burning at the tip of the penis when you urinate?	¿Alguna vez ha tenido ardor en la punta del pene cuando orina?	¿Alguna vez ha tenido quemazón en la punta del pene al orinar?	
A. No. I have had no burning when I go to the bathroom.	No. No he tenido ardor cuando voy al baño.	No.	
Q. Do you have to get up at night to go to the bathroom?	¿Tiene que levantarse durante la noche para ir al baño?	¿Tiene que levantarse en la noche a orinar?	
A. Yes. I get up two or three times a night to urinate.	Sí, me levanto dos o tres veces en la noche a orinar.	Sí, me levanto dos o tres veces en la noche.	
Q. Have you had any fever or chills?	¿Ha tenido fiebre o escalofríos?	¿Ha tenido calentura o escalofríos?	
A. Yes. For the past day I have felt warm and have chills.	Sí. Desde ayer me he sentido afiebrado y he tenido escalofríos.	Sí, desde ayer he estado con calentura y con "calofríos".	
Q. Have you had any stomach or back pain?	¿Ha tenido dolor de estómago o de espalda?	¿Le ha dolido el estómago o la espalda?	
A. Yes. It hurts in the lower part of my stomach.	Sí. Me duele en la parte de abajo del estómago.	Sí, me duele el estómago, en la parte de abajo.	

	English	Spanish Formal	Spanish Informal
Q.	Where does it hurt exactly?	¿Dónde le duele exactamente?	¿En qué parte le duele exactamente?
A.	It hurts in the center of my stomach, low down.	Me duele en el centro del estómago, para abajo.	El dolor es en el centro del estómago, abajo.
Q.	Is it constant or does it come and go?	¿Es constante o le va y le viene?	¿Lo tiene todo el tiempo o le pega y se le quita?
A.	It comes and goes.	Viene y se va.	Me pega y se me quita.
Q.	How would you describe the pain?	¿Cómo describiría el dolor?	¿Cómo es el dolor?
A.	It is like a constant pressure.	Es como una presión constante.	Es como una presión que no se quita.
Q.	Does it move anywhere?	¿Se mueve para alguna otra parte del cuerpo?	¿Se le mueve?
A.	No. It stays right in the center of my stomach, low down.	No. Se queda en el centro del estómago, en la parte de abajo.	No.
Q.	Is it getting worse?	¿Está empeorando?	¿Es peor ahora?
A.	Yes. It feels much worse.	Sí, está empeorando.	Sí, es peor ahora.
Q.	What makes it better or worse?	¿Qué lo hace mejor y qué lo hace peor?	¿Qué lo empeora y qué lo mejora?
A.	Nothing really. When I push on this area the pain is much worse.	Realmente nada. Cuando pongo presión en esta área, el dolor es peor.	Nada. Cuando aprieto en esta parte es peor.
Q.	Do you have any medical illnesses such as diabetes, high blood pressure, heart disease, or lung disease?	¿Tiene alguna otra enfermedad como diabetes, presión alta, enfermedad del corazón o de los pulmones?	¿Padece de alguna otra enfermedad, como de la diabetes, la presión alta, el corazón o los pulmones?
A.	I have high blood pressure and take Diovan for that. Otherwise, I am in good health.	Tengo la presión alta y tomo Diovan para eso. Por lo demás, tengo buena salud.	Padezco de la presión alta y tomo Diovan. Pero eso es todo.
Q.	Do you suffer from any nerve or neurologic diseases?	¿Padece de alguna enfermedad neurológica o de los nervios?	¿Tiene alguna enfermedad neurológica o de los nervios?
A.	No, I have no neurologic diseases.	No, no tengo ninguna enfermedad neurológica.	No.
Q.	Do you have any allergies to medications?	¿Es alérgico a algún medicamento?	¿Padece de alergia a alguna medicina?
A.	No, I have no allergies.	No, no tengo alergias.	No.
Q.	Have you ever had surgery before?	¿Alguna vez le han hecho cirugía?	¿Alguna vez lo han operado?
A.	I had my tonsils out as a kid. I also had surgery on my knee when I was about 30 years old.	Me quitaron las amígdalas cuando era pequeño. También me operaron la rodilla cuando tenía como treinta años.	Me sacaron las glándulas cuando era niño. También me operaron de la rodilla cuando tenía treinta años.
Q.	Are you taking any medications besides the Diovan?	¿Está tomando alguna otra medicina, además de Diovan?	Aparte de Diovan, ¿toma alguna otra medicina?
A.	No. I occasionally take ibuprofen when my knee acts up.	No, a veces tomo ibuprofen cuando me molesta la rodilla.	No, de vez en cuando tomo ibuprofen cuando me duele la rodilla.
Q.	Mr. Ortiz, can you change into a gown and I will be right back to do a physical exam.	Sr. Ortiz, ¿se puede poner esta bata? Yo regresaré en un momento para hacerle un examen físico.	Sr. Ortiz, ¿se puede poner esta bata? Regresaré en un momento para examinarlo.

PHYSICAL EXAM

Physical exam is crucial. A complete exam should be done in view of the older age of this patient. Of key importance is the rectal exam, during which one can assess the size of the prostate and its characteristics.

	English	Spanish Formal	Spanish Informal
Q.	Mr. Ortiz, I am going to do a complete exam. This will include a rectal exam so I can examine the prostate.	Sr. Ortiz, le voy a hacer un examen completo. Esto incluye un tacto rectal para poder examinar la próstata.	Sr. Ortiz, le voy a hacer un examen completo, incluyendo un tacto rectal para examinar la próstata.
A.	OK.	Está bien.	Bien.

Of note in the physical exam is the following:

- Temp. 38.5°C, P 98, RR 14, BP 110/70.

- Abdominal exam: Mildly distended. Fullness is noted in the suprapubic region. Bowel sounds are normal to auscultation. Percussion reveals dullness over the suprapubic region. Fullness is noted in the suprapubic region to palpation as well as tenderness. No voluntary or involuntary guarding is present.

- Prostate exam: Smooth, markedly enlarged, non-tender.

Of number one importance is the hypotension and tachycardia exhibited by this patient. Accompanied by the fever, these are signs of septic shock. The fact that our patient is oriented tells us this is most likely early; however, the first order of priority is giving this patient intravenous fluid.

It is apparent by the history that our patient has a problem with his urinary stream. However, although BPH can present with the above symptoms, one has to rule out other causes of impediment to urinary flow. Prostatitis, an infection of the prostate gland, can present with urinary obstruction and fever. Bladder pathology such as tumor or bladder calculi can obstruct outflow of urine. In addition, urethral stricture from repeated infections such as gonorrhea, trauma or prior instrumentation of the urethra for diagnostic purposes may result in urethral stricture, again blocking outflow of urine. A history of neurologic disease may key one into the diagnosis of neurogenic bladder, a disease that causes bladder retention of urine due to problems in bladder contraction. Finally, medications such as antihistamines, which impair bladder function, and alpha-agonists, which impair outflow at the junction of the urethra and bladder due to sphincter contraction, are common precipitators of urinary obstruction, especially in older male patients.

The above findings are consistent with BPH. The fact that the prostate is non-tender makes prostatitis, an infection of the prostate gland, unlikely. The smoothness of the prostate makes prostate cancer less likely but doesn't rule it out 100%. The fever in the presence of urinary retention and a non-tender prostate has to make one think of a secondary urinary tract infection due to the blockage of urine. Due to the obstruction, residual urine is left in the bladder after urination. Normally, less than 20 cc of urine is left in the bladder after voiding. If a large volume of residual urine is left in the bladder following voiding, there is a high risk of secondary infection of this stagnant urine. The palpation of a suprapubic mass, which is dull to percussion, confirms the presence of an overly distended bladder.

Lab tests: A urine analysis and culture is important to diagnose a urinary tract infection, if present. A blood culture should also be done to see if septicemia is present, as well as a complete blood count to look for infection (elevated WBC). A prostate-specific antigen (PSA) should be drawn. This is a sensitive test for prostate cancer, but it is not specific. Results may be elevated in BPH, urinary retention, and prostatitis. If it is elevated in our patient, we should repeat the test when the urinary retention resolves.

A complete set of electrolytes and blood for creatinine and blood urea nitrogen should also be drawn to assess renal function. With urinary retention the kidney may suffer temporary or permanent injury, especially if long-standing uropathy is present.

Next, a Foley catheter should be placed through the urethra to drain the distended bladder. If placement is difficult due to the enlarged prostate, the urologist on call should be consulted immediately. Forced attempt at Foley catheter placement can result in injury to the urethra.

FOLLOW-UP

	English	Spanish Formal	Spanish Informal
Q.	Mr. Ortiz, based on the history and physical exam, I believe you have an enlarged prostate. As a person gets older, the prostate slowly enlarges. The bladder is blocked by the prostate, so no urine comes out. The urine is probably infected, based on your fever and low blood pressure. The first step is to give you intravenous fluids and antibiotics and then drain the bladder. To do this, we put a tube in the bladder through the tip of the penis, the urethra. We will numb that up with a jelly before inserting the tube. That will make you feel much better. We will also draw some blood and check the urine for infection of the urine and blood. We will give you antibiotics through your vein to control the infection. You need to be admitted to the hospital and the urologist will see you in the hospital to discuss how to manage this enlarged prostate. Medications can be used, and in some cases surgery is used to cut part of the prostate out to relieve the blockage. Do you have any questions?	Sr. Ortiz, de acuerdo con la historia y el examen físico, yo creo que usted tiene la próstata aumentada de tamaño. La próstata crece lentamente conforme la persona va envejeciendo. La vejiga esta obstruida por la próstata, por lo que la orina no puede salir. Por la fiebre y la baja presión arterial, es probable que la orina esté infectada. El primer paso es darle fluidos intravenosos y antibióticos, y después drenar la vejiga. Para hacerlo, le vamos a colocar una sonda en la vejiga a través de la uretra. Le vamos a dormir esa parte con una jalea antes de insertar la sonda. Se sentirá mucho mejor. También le vamos a sacar algo de sangre y examinar la orina para ver si hay infección en la orina y la sangre. Le vamos a dar antibióticos por la vena para controlar la infección. Vamos a tener que internarlo en el hospital y el urólogo lo va a ver para discutir la mejor manera de tratar el crecimiento de la próstata. En algunos casos se pueden usar medicamentos, mientras en otros se usa cirugía para quitar una parte de la próstata y aliviar la obstrucción. ¿Tiene alguna pregunta?	Sr. Ortiz, yo creo que usted tiene un crecimiento de la próstata. La próstata crece poco a poco, conforme la persona va envejeciendo. La vejiga está bloqueada por la próstata, por lo que la orina no puede salir. Por la fiebre y la presión baja, es posible que exista una infección. Lo primero es darle líquidos por la vena y ponerle antibióticos, después le vamos a sacar la orina de la vejiga. Para esto, le vamos a meter una sonda en la vejiga a través de la uretra. Le vamos a dormir esa parte con una jalea antes de meter la sonda. Se sentirá mejor. También le vamos a sacar sangre y examinar la orina para ver si hay infección. Le daremos antibióticos por la vena para controlar la infección. Hay que internarlo en el hospital y el urólogo lo vendrá a ver para discutir la mejor manera de tratar su problema. A veces se puede tratar con medicinas. Otras veces hay que operar para quitar una parte de la próstata y aliviar el bloqueo. ¿Tiene preguntas?
A.	Is it cancer?	¿Es cáncer?	¿Es cáncer?

English	Spanish Formal	Spanish Informal	Continued
Q. We will draw some blood to look to see if the prostate has cancer. The test is called PSA. However, it is sometimes abnormal when the prostate is big and blocks the urine, so it might need to be repeated. Most likely this is benign, not cancer.	Vamos a sacarle sangre para ver si la próstata tiene cáncer. El examen se llama PSA (antígeno prostático específico). Sin embargo, a veces es anormal cuando la próstata está agrandada y hay obstrucción de orina, por lo que puede ser necesario repetirla. Posiblemente esto es benigno y no un cáncer.	Vamos a hacerle un examen de sangre que se llama PSA para ver si hay cáncer. El examen a veces es anormal cuando la próstata está aumentada de tamaño, por lo que puede ser necesario repetirlo. Posiblemente es benigno y no un cáncer.	

VOCABULARY

English	Español
Benign prostatic hypertrophy (BPH)	Hipertrofia prostática benigna, padecer de la próstata
Bladder cancer	Cáncer de la vejiga
Blood urea nitrogen (BUN)	Nitrógeno úrico en sangre
Catheter	Catéter, sonda
Creatinine clearance test	Prueba de aclaramiento de creatinina
Cryptorchism	Criptorquidia, criptorquismo
Cystectomy	Cistectomía, operación para remover la vejiga
Cystitis	Cistitis, infección de la vejiga, mal de orín
Cystocele	Cistocele
Cystoscopy	Cistoscopía, endoscopía de la vejiga
Dialysis	Diálisis
Dysuria	Disuria, ardor al orinar, dolor al orinar, dificultad para orinar
Enuresis	Enuresis, no orinar
Epididymitis	Epididimitis, inflamación del epidídimo
Glomerulonephritis	Glomerulonefritis, inflamación del tejido de los riñones
Glycosuria	Glicosuria, orina con azúcar
Hematuria	Hematuria, orina con sangre
Hydronephrosis	Hidronefrosis
Inguinal hernia	Hernia inguinal
Intravenous pyelogram	Pielograma intravenoso, estudio radiográfico de las vías urinarias
Lithotripsy	Litotripsia
Nephrolithiasis	Nefrolitiasis, cálculos o piedras de los riñones
Nephrotic syndrome	Síndrome nefrótico

English	Español
Nocturia	Nocturia, levantarse a orinar en la noche, después de acostarse
Oliguria	Oliguria, orinar menos de lo normal
Polycystic kidneys	Riñones poliquísticos
Polyuria	Poliuria, orinar mucho, orinadera
Prostate	Próstata
Prostatitis	Prostatitis, inflamación de la próstata
Pyuria	Piuria, orina con pus
Renal angiography	Angiografía renal
Renal calculi	Cálculos renales, piedras en el riñón
Renal colic	Cólico renal
Renal failure	Insuficiencia renal
Retrograde pyelogram	Pielograma retrógrado
Vesical tenesmus	Tenesmo vesical, ganas urgentes de orinar que obligan a la persona a orinar frecuentemente
Urea	Urea
Ureters	Uréteres
Urethra	Uretra
Urethritis	Uretritis, inflamación de la uretra
Uric acid	Ácido úrico
Urinalysis	Examen de orina
Urinary incontinence	Incontinencia urinaria
Urinary retention	Retención urinaria
Urology	Urología
Uterus	Útero, matriz
Vesicoureteral reflux	Reflujo vesicoureteral

GRAMMATICAL TIPS

FUTURE TENSE

The future tense is triggered when expressing facts yet to take place. Since the future is a probability, it also includes an aspect called the conditional. In English, the future is indicated by the auxiliary verb will. For example, telling a patient, "You will take two tablets every day." In Spanish, the future is formed with its proper endings and using the verb in the infinitive as follows:

	Hablar	Comer	Vivir
Yo	hablaré	comeré	viviré
Tú	hablarás	comerás	vivirás
Él, Ella, Usted	hablará	comerá	vivirá
Nosotros	hablaremos	comeremos	viviremos
Ellos, Ellas, Ustedes	hablarán	comerán	vivirán

Notice that the endings for the conjugations of the verbs are exactly the same.

Here is a list of irregular verbs in the future and conditional tenses. For irregular verbs, the only change is in the stem, not in the endings. The endings are the same as the regular verbs.

Poner	Pondr-	Caber	Cabr-
Valer	Valdr-	Poder	Podr-
Tener	Tendr-	Saber	Sabr-
Salir	Saldr-	Hacer	Har-
Querer	Querr-	Decir	Dir-

Ejercicios Con El Futuro De Verbos Irregulares:

The conditional is used with probability when an action was supposed to occur and did not occur: "He said she would be here tonight," and when a condition has to be met for such an action to happen: "If I were a doctor, I would cure many illnesses."

As said previously, the conditional is an aspect of the future tense and the conjugation is done with the endings *ía, ías, ía, íamos, ían.*

For example:

	Hablar	Comer	Vivir
Yo	hablaría	comería	viviría
Tú	hablarías	comerías	vivirías
Él, Ella, Usted	hablaría	comería	viviría
Nosotros	hablaríamos	comeríamos	viviríamos
Ellos, Ellas, Ustedes	hablarían	comerían	vivirían

Futuro simple

Completa las siguientes frases empleando el futuro de los verbos que aparecen entre paréntesis:

1. Él _____ (*ir*) a hacerse un chequeo general al hospital.

2. Ellos nos _____ (*invitar*) a comer en la cafetería.

3. Las enfermeras no_____ (*comer*) en la cafetería porque no les gusta ese lugar.

CULTURAL TIPS: NATURE

Within some of the indigenous cultures, nature has unlimited power. The moon, the sun, and the stars have an effect on the earth and on humans. There is a period during the summer when it is believed that the earth cleanses itself. Since we have lost much of our sensitivity to the earth, we are not aware or sensitive to this period, but we are affected by it. The *canícula* is such a period. During this time, the earth releases a sort of toxin that is absorbed by plants. The plants are eaten by humans and animals, so we are consuming the toxins. These toxins cause stomach or digestive problems. Sometimes we see animals eating grass to cleanse themselves when they feel uncomfortable. As humans, we have lost such sensitivity to this period; nonetheless, we suffer a lot of digestive problems during the summer.

The sun and the moon also have a direct effect on the earth. People in some native cultures believe that when there is an eclipse, a strong energy exerts an effect. An eclipse can either add or remove parts of what a normal piece or being can be. For example, when there is a lunar eclipse, it is believed that it will result in a missing body part. In consequence, sometimes we see a malformation and it is believed that it is caused by the lunar eclipse. To prevent malformation not only in plants but in babies, pregnant women tie a piece of red cloth or fabric around their wrists during the gestation period. It is believed that the most vulnerable state is when the baby is developing. When babies are born with a cleft pallet, the mothers will feel guilty. Some farmers will tie this piece of red fabric to trees to protect them from the eclipse and avoid damage to their crops. When there is a solar eclipse, the opposite occurs. The sun is believed to add parts and pregnant women must wear something made out of gold to prevent damage to the fetus. These beliefs are very strong among some native cultures of Latin America.

Index

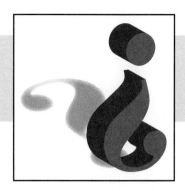

Note: Page numbers followed by f refer to figures